YOUR GUIDE TO

CANCER PREVENTION

Edited by
Joni L. Watson, MBA, MSN, RN, OCN®

Oncology Nursing Society
Pittsburgh, Pennsylvania

ONS Publications Department
Publisher and Director of Publications: William A. Tony, BA, CQIA
Senior Editorial Manager: Lisa M. George, BA
Assistant Editorial Manager: Amy Nicoletti, BA, JD
Acquisitions Editor: John Zaphyr, BA, MEd
Associate Staff Editors: Casey S. Kennedy, BA, Andrew Petyak, BA
Design and Production Administrator: Dany Sjoen
Editorial Assistant: Judy Holmes

Library of Congress Cataloging-in-Publication Data
Names: Watson, Joni L., editor.
Title: Your guide to cancer prevention / edited by Joni L. Watson, MBA, MSN, RN, OCN.
Description: Pittsburgh, Pennsylvania : Oncology Nursing Society, [2018] | Includes bibliographical references. |
Identifiers: LCCN 2017043807 (print) | LCCN 2017044591 (ebook) | ISBN 9781635930139 () | ISBN 9781635930122 (paperback)
Subjects: LCSH: Cancer–Prevention–Popular works.
Classification: LCC RC268 (ebook) | LCC RC268 .Y69 2018 (print) | DDC 616.99/4052–dc23
LC record available at https://lccn.loc.gov/2017043807

Publisher's Note
This book is published by the Oncology Nursing Society (ONS). ONS neither represents nor guarantees that the practices described herein will, if followed, ensure safe and effective patient care. The recommendations contained in this book reflect ONS's judgment regarding the state of general knowledge and practice in the field as of the date of publication. The recommendations may not be appropriate for use in all circumstances. Those who use this book should make their own determinations regarding specific safe and appropriate patient care practices, taking into account the personnel, equipment, and practices available at the hospital or other facility at which they are located. The editor and publisher cannot be held responsible for any liability incurred as a consequence from the use or application of any of the contents of this book. Figures and tables are used as examples only. They are not meant to be all-inclusive, nor do they represent endorsement of any particular institution by ONS. Mention of specific products and opinions related to those products do not indicate or imply endorsement by ONS. Websites mentioned are provided for information only; the hosts are responsible for their own content and availability. Unless otherwise indicated, dollar amounts reflect U.S. dollars.

ONS publications are originally published in English. Publishers wishing to translate ONS publications must contact ONS about licensing arrangements. ONS publications cannot be translated without obtaining written permission from ONS. (Individual tables and figures that are reprinted or adapted require additional permission from the original source.) Because translations from English may not always be accurate or precise, ONS disclaims any responsibility for inaccuracies in words or meaning that may occur as a result of the translation. Readers relying on precise information should check the original English version.

Printed in the United States of America

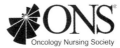

Oncology Nursing Society

Innovation • Excellence • Advocacy

Contributors

Editor

Joni L. Watson, MBA, MSN, RN, OCN®
Director, Operations
Baylor Scott and White Hillcrest Medical Center
Waco, Texas

Authors

Deborah Christensen, MSN, RN,
AOCNS®, HNB-BC
Oncology Nurse Navigator
Southwest Cancer Center
St. George, Utah
Chapter 2. Sun Safety

Stella Dike, MSN, RN, OCN®
Nurse Educator
University of Texas MD Anderson Cancer
Center
Houston, Texas
Chapter 11. Cancer and the Environment

Kristin Shea Donahue, RN, MSN, OCN®
Director of Educational Services
Clearview Cancer Institute
Huntsville, Alabama
Chapter 3. Screening for Cancer

Colleen H. Erb, MSN, CRNP, ACNP-BC,
AOCNP®
Nurse Practitioner, Hematology-
Oncology
Abramson Cancer Center, Hospital of the
University of Pennsylvania
Philadelphia, Pennsylvania
Chapter 7. Viruses and Vaccines

Katrina Fetter, MSN, RN, AOCNS®,
AGCNS-BC
Oncology Clinical Nurse Specialist
Lancaster General Health/Penn Medicine
Lancaster, Pennsylvania
Chapter 4. Physical Activity

Andrew S. Guinigundo, MSN, RN, CNP,
ANP-BC
Lead Advanced Practice Provider, Nurse
Practitioner
Oncology Hematology Care, Inc.
Cincinnati, Ohio
Chapter 6. Alcohol and Tobacco

Kelsey Haley, MSN, RN, OCN®
Professional Development Specialist,
   Oncology
Baylor Scott and White Health
Dallas, Texas
*Chapter 8. Physiologic Stress and
Inflammation; Chapter 9. Radiation
Exposure*

Tina Henderson, MPH, CHSP
Manager, Environmental Health and
   Safety
University of Texas MD Anderson Cancer
   Center
Houston, Texas
Chapter 11. Cancer and the Environment

Tiffiny Jackson, RN, MS, FNP-BC
Nurse Practitioner
Lyda Hill Cancer Prevention Center
University of Texas MD Anderson Cancer
   Center
Houston, Texas
Chapter 11. Cancer and the Environment

**Suzanne M. Mahon, RN, DNSc, AOCN®,
   AGN-BC**
Professor, Internal Medicine, Division of
   Hematology and Oncology
Professor, Adult Nursing, School of
   Nursing
Saint Louis University
St. Louis, Missouri
Chapter 10. Genetics

**Marlon G. Saria, PhD, RN, AOCNS®,
   FAAN**
Assistant Professor and Director, Center
   for Quality and Outcomes Research
Pacific Neuroscience Institute and John
   Wayne Cancer Institute at Providence
   Saint John's Health Center
Santa Monica, California
Chapter 1. Overview of Cancer

Jane Taylor Williams, MSN, RN, FNP-BC
Advanced Practice Provider
University of Texas MD Anderson Cancer
   Center
Houston, Texas
Chapter 5. Food and Nutrition

Disclosure

Editors and authors of books and guidelines provided by the Oncology Nursing Society are expected to disclose to the readers any significant financial interest or other relationships with the manufacturer(s) of any commercial products.

A vested interest may be considered to exist if a contributor is affiliated with or has a financial interest in commercial organizations that may have a direct or indirect interest in the subject matter. A "financial interest" may include, but is not limited to, being a shareholder in the organization; being an employee of the commercial organization; serving on an organization's speakers bureau; or receiving research funding from the organization. An "affiliation" may be holding a position on an advisory board or some other role of benefit to the commercial organization. Vested interest statements appear in the front matter for each publication.

Contributors are expected to disclose any unlabeled or investigational use of products discussed in their content. This information is acknowledged solely for the information of the readers.

The contributors provided the following disclosure and vested interest information:
Joni L. Watson, MBA, MSN, RN, OCN®: Oncology Nursing Society, leadership position; Oncology Nursing Society, Tesaro, Inc., honoraria
Deborah Christensen, MSN, RN, AOCNS®, HNB-BC: Takeda Pharmaceutical Company Ltd, consultant or advisory role; Academy of Oncology Nurse Navigators, Takeda Pharmaceutical Company Ltd, honoraria

Kristin Shea Donahue, RN, MSN, OCN®: Genentech, Inc., consultant or advisory role

Andrew S. Guinigundo, MSN, RN, CNP, ANP-BC: Amgen Inc., Genentech, Inc., consultant or advisory role; Amgen Inc., Astellas Pharma US, Inc., Celgene Corporation, Genentech, Inc., Merck & Co., Inc., Pfizer Inc., honoraria

Marlon G. Saria, PhD, RN, AOCNS®, FAAN: Brain Cancer Research Institute, John Wayne Cancer Institute, San Diego Brain Tumor Foundation, U.S. Department of the Air Force, leadership positions; CancerLife, consultant; ICU Medical, Inc., honoraria

Contents

Preface

An ounce of prevention is worth a pound of cure.
—Benjamin Franklin

Far too many of my loved ones and those I have had the privilege to care for have lost their lives to the group of diseases we generally think of as one disease—cancer. As an oncology nurse, I have devoted my life to caring for people affected by cancer; this book is an extension of that care. The American Institute for Cancer Research estimates one-third of all cancers are preventable, and the World Health Organization suggests upwards of half of all cancers are preventable, meaning they would not occur with a healthy lifestyle and screening changes. How incredible to think we hold in our hands the power to prevent many cancers. What power to care for ourselves and those we love most. This book holds such power—information on ounces of cancer prevention.

Thirteen oncology nurses have gathered cancer prevention evidence and tools for you. The following chapters discuss both modifiable cancer risk factors (those we have the immediate power and control to change, such as nutrition and physical activity) as well as nonmodifiable risk factors (those we have no control over, such as age, gender, ethnicity, and heredity). Oncology nurses specifically curated the appendices with you in mind, and they include helpful resources (Appendix A), practical cancer screening tools (Appendix B), and references (Appendix C)— the weighty evidence—supporting all statements. Each chapter also includes a glossary to break down scientific and medical jargon. When a word is bolded in the text, you can learn more by seeing the glossary at the end of the chapter.

As with the ever-developing world of cancer care, cancer prevention is always changing thanks to trained, dedicated researchers in many fields of study. Because of this innovation, take special caution to talk with your healthcare providers about your health, modifiable cancer risk factors, and cancer screening recommendations, as information may have changed since the publication of this book.

Chapter by chapter—ounce by ounce—you can help prevent cancer.

Joni L. Watson, MBA, MSN, RN, OCN®

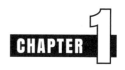

CHAPTER 1

Overview of Cancer

Marlon G. Saria, PhD, RN, AOCNS®, FAAN

I will also ask for an appropriation of an extra $100 million to launch an intensive campaign to find a cure for cancer, and I will ask later for whatever additional funds can effectively be used. The time has come in America when the same kind of concentrated effort that split the atom and took man to the moon should be turned toward conquering this dread disease. Let us make a total national commitment to achieve this goal. America has long been the wealthiest nation in the world. Now it is time we became the healthiest nation in the world.
—President Richard Nixon,
State of the Union Address, January 22, 1971

For the loved ones we've all lost, for the families that we can still save, let's make America the country that cures cancer once and for all.
—President Barack Obama,
State of the Union Address, January 12, 2016

How can one word evoke such powerful emotions that range from disinterest to panic, from sadness to a firm determination to defy and overcome? Cancer survivor Gwen Andrews Nacos, founder of Cedars CanSupport, described

1

the far-reaching impact of cancer when she said, "Cancer is not just a diagnosis. It becomes a way of life. When a person is diagnosed with cancer, the whole family gets cancer." Many factors can increase the chances of cancer showing up uninvited at our front doors. Some of these factors we can't do anything about—called *nonmodifiable risk factors*—while other factors we can change to lessen our risk of developing cancer. To combat the disease, cancer care is a threefold strategy: prevent cancer cases that can be prevented, cure all that can be cured, and manage the symptoms when a cure is not possible.

Although cancer is still the second leading cause of death in the United States, progress in cancer research is improving survival. Today, more people with cancer are living at least five years after a diagnosis than in the 1970s. It was not until 1937, when President Franklin Delano Roosevelt launched the National Cancer Institute (NCI), that we started to build the foundation of our knowledge on the causes and treatments of cancer. Surgery and radiation therapy were being used in the treatment of cancer even before the creation of NCI, yet their success was limited to individual cases. We got our first glimpse of improved outcomes for populations in 1943 when the Pap test led to dramatic declines in cervical cancer deaths and reduction in U.S. cervical cancer rates by 70%.

FACT OR FICTION? Cancer is a recent disease caused by our Western customs.

Fiction. Cancer is not a disease of the modern world. It has been described in ancient texts as early as 3000 BC, and evidence of the disease has been found in fossilized bone tumors.

In cancer treatment, the role of chemotherapy gained wide popularity in 1947 through the landmark case of a four-year-old girl with leukemia, the first known response of pediatric leukemia to a chemotherapy drug. It would be another two years before the

U.S. Food and Drug Administration approved the first chemotherapy drug for the treatment of cancer, nitrogen mustard.

Like its wide array of treatments, *cancer* is a broad term often used to describe a large group of diseases defined by uncontrolled cell growth and division. It is important to emphasize that cancer is not one but many individual diseases that share a few key characteristics yet are distinct from each other. The following characteristics define cancer:

- Uncontrolled proliferation—Cancer cells can grow out of control and form new tissue.
- Abnormal differentiation—Cancer cells do not mature normally; therefore, they are not able to carry out their functions.
- Loss of **apoptosis**—Cancer cells do not follow the typical cell cycle that leads to programmed cell death.
- Loss of contact inhibition—Cancer cells ignore signals to stop dividing, and they do not die off to keep the number of cells constant.
- Loss of cohesiveness and adhesiveness—Cancer cells can break away from the mass of cells, circulate through blood and **lymphatic** vessels, and spread to distant sites.
- Impaired cellular communication—Cancer cells do not wait for signals from the body to form new tissue.
- Tumor markers—Cancer cells can express (or overexpress) proteins, called *antigens*, on the cell surface, which makes them different from normal, healthy cells.

It only takes one cell to transform (or *mutate*) and grow out of control for cancer to develop. This continued cell division leads to the growth of solid lumps in any part of the body—in any of the organs or tissues in the body (*solid cancers*) or an increase in any of the components of the blood cells (*hematologic* or *blood cancers*). Cancer can affect people of any age but occurs more often in older people, most likely from cumulative exposure to **carcinogens**, agents that are known to increase cancer risk. Cancer comes from our own cells; however, our chances of being affected by the disease can be linked to factors that come from both within and outside of our bodies. Risks can be driven by genetic predisposition or environmental and lifestyle factors. For most people who develop cancer, mutations happen at random (known as *sporadic mutation*); however, a small percentage of cancers will occur in individuals with an inherited mutation (referred to as *hereditary cancer*).

How Cancer Develops

Carcinogenesis or *oncogenesis* is the process by which normal cells transform into cancerous, or **malignant**, cells. Development of cancer is a complex process that, despite decades of research, we still do not completely understand. One of the most common explanations is that no single event directly leads to cancer occurring. According to multiple sources, a series of processes cause normal cells to change into malignant cells.

Most healthy cells follow an internal clock, what is commonly referred to as the *cell cycle*, meaning they go through stages in life. The cell cycle begins when a single cell divides into two daughter cells. The progression of the cell cycle is regulated by signals from outside and within the cells. Interrupting or altering these signals can lead to changes within the cells.

The three-stage theory of carcinogenesis is one of the most common explanations for the development of cancer. This theory divides cancer development into three stages: initiation, **promotion**, and **progression**. The theory is largely used for teaching purposes, as it is limited by the lack of biologic markers that define each of the stages.

Initiation

Initiation, the first stage, is when initial cell mutation occurs. It may involve one or more cellular changes that are either spontaneous or started by exposure to a carcinogen. These changes create a potential for the affected cell and its daughter cells to develop into a cancer cell. A disruption in the cell development cycle can be caused by a response to the activation of cellular genes known as *oncogenes*, the portion of **deoxyribonucleic acid** (DNA) that regulates normal cell growth and repair. Inactivation, on the other hand, is the process whereby cellular genes known as *tumor suppressor genes* alter the normal cell cycle. Tumor suppressor genes are the components of DNA that stop, inhibit, or suppress cell division. Mutations in oncogenes and tumor suppressor genes allow cells to grow beyond normal body needs. The new cell clones that arise from the cellular changes typically have a selective and reproductive advantage over the original cells. The new cells exhibit uncontrolled division and loss of what is called *apoptosis,* or *programmed cell death. Apoptotic genes* are the components of DNA that control cell death. Mutations in apoptotic genes allow cancer cells to evade cell death.

FACT OR FICTION: Cancer cells can live forever.

Fact. Scientists have found a way to keep cancer cells immortal. HeLa cells are an "immortal cell line" used widely in cancer laboratories around the world. Considered the oldest human cancer cell line, the first HeLa cells were taken from the cervix of patient Henrietta Lacks on February 8, 1951. The cultured offspring cells have since been used in many scientific efforts, including cancer therapies, AIDS treatment, genetic mapping, and vaccine development, to name a few.

Promotion

Promotion is the second stage where the transformed (or *initiated*) cells are stimulated to divide. The environment within (*intracellular*) and outside (*extracellular*) the cell influences cancer development. Malignant transformation may involve more than one step and requires repeated exposures to promoting agents. For example, one tumor promoter is estrogen, a naturally occurring hormone that by itself will not "initiate" cancer. However, estrogen can drive the growth of a mutated breast cell.

Progression

Progression is the third stage in the three-stage theory of cancer causation. During progression, tumor cells compete with one another to survive, leading to more mutations that make the cells more aggressive. As the tumor increases in size, the cells undergo further mutations, leading to increased *heterogeneity* within the tumor. *Heterogeneity* refers to multiple genetic variants of the mutated or transformed cell. With increased heterogeneity, the cancer cells found in one lump or mass can look and act differently, making diagnosis and treatment increasingly harder.

Tumor Metastasis

Cancer cells are distinct in that they have lost important features of normal cells, one of which is adhesiveness. Molecules on a normal cell surface allow them to bind to other cells with similar molecules, so when cellular adhesiveness exists, normal cells literally stick together and stay in the right place within the body.

Cancer cells, however, lose these adhesive molecules. As a result, cancer cells can easily break away from their neighbors and invade other tissues, which is known as *metastasis*, the primary cause of cancer spreading to other organs and tissues. Additionally, rogue cells can also enter the blood and lymphatic vessels and be transported to more distant sites within the body.

Cancer Risk Factors

Many known or suspected biologic or environmental factors are associated with the development of cancer. Biologic factors we cannot control include age, gender, family history, and genetic predisposition. Environmental factors that can be controlled include diet, weight, radiation and sunlight exposure, tobacco use, infections (viruses), and exposure to chemicals, such as asbestos, dyes, and food additives. Although it is highly recommended to prevent or avoid the risk factors that can lead to cancer, it is not always possible to do so. Early detection is key in the treatment of cancers related to nonmodifiable risk factors.

Age and Gender

Cancer has long been associated with increasing age. While no age group is immune to cancer, evidence has shown that cancers are found more frequently in people aged 50 and older. NCI found that between 1975 and 2013, about 1,300 in every 100,000 people aged 50 and older were diagnosed with cancer each year. During the same time frame, NCI found about 100 in every 100,000 people younger than age 50 were diagnosed with cancer.

The role of hormones has been established in gender-specific cancers (breast, endometrial, ovarian, prostate, and testicular), thyroid cancer, and bone cancer. According to a 2000 study by Henderson and Feigelson, these cancers account for more than 35% of all newly diagnosed cancers in men and more than 40% of all newly diagnosed cancers in women.

Sunlight

Exposure to ultraviolet rays from the sun, sunlamps, and tanning booths has been linked to skin cancer. Chapter 2 shares more information on ultraviolet light as well as how to reduce exposure.

Physical Activity, Diet, and Obesity

Maintaining a healthy weight is an important way to reduce overall cancer risk, as obesity is linked to several cancers. Although multiple studies have compared the diets of people with and without cancer, very few have shown that any specific component causes cancer or protects against cancer. In other words, these results only show a link, not a specific cause. Obesity has been associated with an increased risk for many types of cancer, including breast, colorectal, endometrial, esophageal, kidney, pancreatic, and gallbladder. Chapter 4 delves into physical activity and its protective mechanisms, while Chapter 5 discusses food and nutrition in more detail.

Tobacco and Alcohol

Tobacco use is the leading cause of cancer. There is no safe level of tobacco use. Tobacco is linked to lung, esophageal, bladder, kidney, stomach, colorectal, and cervical cancers, among others. Alcohol consumption is also linked to several cancers. Use of both alcohol and tobacco further increases risk. Chapter 6 discusses these largely modifiable cancer risk factors in detail.

Viruses and Infections

Some viruses can cause cancer. Human papillomavirus (commonly known as HPV) can cause cervical cancer; Epstein-Barr virus can cause non-Hodgkin lymphoma; hepatitis B virus can cause liver cancer; and human T-cell leukemia virus can cause leukemia. In addition to viruses, bacteria and parasites have also been associated with certain cancers. *Helicobacter pylori* (*H. pylori*) is a type of bacteria that can cause stomach cancer, and *Schistosoma haematobium*, a flatworm, has been directly associated with bladder cancer. Chapter 7 provides more information on viruses and vaccines.

Stress and Inflammation

Physiologic stress occurs when the body faces a potential or actual threat or demand. Under normal circumstances, stress is a natural occurrence, and in return, the immune system launches an inflammatory response. The inflammatory response is a controlled, protective process that resolves the threat or demand and restores the body's environment for optimal functioning. However, when this process begins or continues inappropriately, damage to the body's cells and genetic material may occur and lead to cancer. Chapter 8 discusses this in more detail.

Radiation

Although radiation is an established carcinogen, lower-energy forms of radiation from electromagnetic fields and mobile phones have not been linked to cancer. Chapter 9 provides more insight on radiation as both a modifiable and nonmodifiable cancer risk factor.

Genetics

Studies focusing on the causes of cancer highlight the relevance of family history as a cancer risk factor. Tools designed to estimate a person's risk of developing a specific cancer consider the number of **first-degree relatives** (parents, siblings, and children) who have been diagnosed with the same cancer. Having a first-degree relative who has been diagnosed with a specific cancer (for example, breast or colorectal cancer) increases a person's risk of developing the same cancer.

NCI reports about 5%–10% of all cancers are attributed to known genetic syndromes. Chapter 10 contains more information about the most common inherited cancer syndromes, the associated genes, and the related cancer types.

Environment

The International Agency for Research on Cancer has identified more than 100 substances as human carcinogens. The National Toxicology Program currently identifies 56 known and 187 "reasonably anticipated" carcinogens. Some of these chemicals include asbestos, benzene, coal-tar pitch, diesel engine exhaust, formaldehyde, leather dust, and soot, among many other common substances. Chapter 11 discusses more of these cancer-causing agents in our everyday environments.

Summary

Cancer describes a group of diseases with one common feature: uncontrolled cell division. All cancers involve a genetic component in that all cancer involves a mutation, but not all cancers are hereditary. Many theories exist on why we develop cancer. One of the most widely used is the three-stage theory of carcinogenesis, which defines cancer development as a complex process that we still do not completely understand. It also describes the association between certain biologic or environmental factors and an increased risk of developing cancer.

Recommended Reading

Amuta, A.O., & Barry, A.E. (2015). Influence of family history of cancer on engagement in protective health behaviors. *American Journal of Health Education, 46,* 157–164. doi:10.1080/19325037.2015.1023478

Anisimov, V.N. (2007). Biology of aging and cancer. *Cancer Control, 14,* 23–31. Retrieved from https://www.ncbi.nlm.nih.gov/pubmed/17242668

Siegel, R.L., Miller, K.D., & Jemal, A. (2017). Cancer statistics, 2017. *CA: A Cancer Journal for Clinicians, 67,* 7–30. doi:10.3322/caac.21387

Skloot, R. (2010). *The immortal life of Henrietta Lacks.* New York, NY: Random House.

Glossary

apoptosis [ap-uh-toh-sis]—A normal, genetically regulated process leading to the death of cells and triggered by the presence or absence of certain stimuli, such as DNA damage.

carcinogen [kahr-sin-uh-jen]—Any substance or agent that tends to produce a cancer.

deoxyribonucleic acid [dee-ok-si-rahy-boh-noo-klee-ik]—An extremely long macromolecule that is the main component of chromosomes and is the material that transfers genetic characteristics in all life forms. Abbreviated as DNA.

extracellular [ek-struh-sel-yuh-ler]—Outside a cell or cells.

first-degree relative—One's mother, father, or biologically related sister(s) or brother(s). People are more likely to share potentially inherited conditions with first-degree relatives than with other more distantly related family members.

intracellular [in-truh-sel-yuh-ler]—Within a cell or cells.

lymphatic [lim-fat-ik]—Pertaining to, containing, or conveying lymph.

malignant [muh-lig-nunt]—Cancerous. Malignant cells can invade and destroy nearby tissue and spread to other parts of the body.

metastasis [meh-tas-tuh-sis]—The spread of cancer cells from the place where they first formed to another part of the body. In metastasis, cancer cells break away from the original (primary) tumor, travel through the blood or lymph system, and form a new tumor in other organs or tissues of the body. The new metastatic tumor is the same type of cancer as the primary tumor. For example, if breast cancer spreads to the lung, the cancer cells in the lung are breast cancer cells, not lung cancer cells. Plural: metastases [meh-tas-tuh-seez].

oncogene [on-koh-jeen]— A mutated form of a gene involved in normal cell growth that may cause the growth of cancer cells. Mutations in genes that become oncogenes can be inherited or caused by exposure to substances in the environment that cause cancer.

progression—In medicine, the course of a disease, such as cancer, as it becomes worse or spreads in the body.

promotion—Stage of carcinogenesis in which initiated cells are prompted to grow and survive.

tumor suppressor gene—A type of gene that makes a protein called a tumor suppressor protein that helps control cell growth. Mutations in tumor suppressor genes may lead to cancer. Also called anti-oncogene.

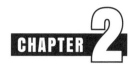

CHAPTER 2

Sun Safety

Deborah Christensen, MSN, RN, AOCNS®, HNB-BC

> *The sun is a wonderful thing, but it can be a very devas-*
> *tating thing.*
>
> —Giada De Laurentiis,
> chef and television host whose
> brother died of melanoma

A day at the beach. Fishing at the lake. A picnic in the park. What do these activities have in common? Bright blue sky and sunshine. Depending on how long you stay in the sun and what protections you use, enjoying a sunny day can be either beneficial or hazardous. The sun's rays, even on a cloudy day, can harm your skin. In general, people with fair skin are more at risk for sun damage than people with darker skin. However, having darker skin pigment does not eliminate the potential for sunburn or skin damage. Your genetic makeup also affects your risk for skin damage and cancer. This chapter discusses sunlight's effect on body tissues, the signs of sun damage and cancerous skin lesions, how to protect your skin, and special safeguards for children, older adults, and people who work outdoors.

Sun Basics

Types of Sunlight

The types of sunlight that pass through the earth's atmosphere are classified based on wavelength. Light that the human eye can see has a longer wavelength than invisible ultraviolet (UV) light, which is divided into three categories—UVA, UVB, and UVC. UVA has the longest wavelength, and UVC has the shortest wavelength. UVA is the most abundant form of UV radiation, and over time, exposure can lead to skin aging and damage. Because of its longer wavelength, UVA penetrates the deeper layers of the skin's surface. The intensity of UVA is the same throughout the day, and clouds or glass surfaces like windows don't block it.

The shorter wavelengths of UVB cause the most damage to the outer layer of the skin and are responsible for the skin reddening and sunburn. In the United States, UVB is the most penetrating from April through October and between the hours of 10 am and 4 pm. Cloud coverage offers some protection from UVB, but it can penetrate through glass, so caution and protection are recommended. The short wavelength of UVC does not reach the earth's surface, so it is of little concern in regard to skin damage.

In general, UV radiation is not inherently bad; it is the length and type of exposure that can produce the harmful effects. Therefore, learning more about the effects of UV rays can help you make healthy choices and balance the risks and benefits of UV exposure.

Vitamin D

Vitamin D production is an important benefit of UVA. When exposed to sunlight, skin cells produce vitamin D, which the liver and kidneys make usable for the body. This nutrient helps with the absorption of calcium and phosphorus from food for bone health. Immune function and blood cell development require adequate levels of vitamin D, yet UV overexposure has also been linked to a decrease in cellular immunity. Food sources naturally rich in vitamin D include fatty fish like salmon, tuna, and sardines. Egg yolks, some types of mushrooms, and ricotta cheese also contain some vitamin D. In addition, dairy products and breakfast cereals are often fortified with vitamin D, so most people in the United States can get adequate vitamin D from fortified foods. Research shows that as little as two to three days of 5–15 minutes of sun exposure to your face, hands, and arms during the summer months can maintain vitamin D levels for most people.

FACT OR FICTION: Wearing sunscreen prevents proper vitamin D production.

Fiction. A 2009 review of the literature found routine and "normal" sunscreen use did not limit vitamin D production to insufficient levels.

UV Overexposure

A significant effect of overexposure to UV light is damage to the DNA of eyes, skin, and body cells—damage that can ultimately lead to cancer. One of the ways you can understand how much UV light is good and how much is harmful is by using the UV index established by the U.S. Environmental Protection Agency (EPA).

UV Index

The UV index is a system used to predict the potential UV exposure at a specific location in the United States. The National Weather Service uses a specialized formula to calculate the UV index. Exposure risk scores range from 0 to 11+ and can be found by using a zip code to specify a location (www.epa.gov/enviro/uv-index-search). Table 2-1 shows the exposure rankings and lists some ways you can protect your skin from sun exposure and damage.

Time of Day, Elevation, and Seasons

The time of day you are exposed to the sun makes a big difference. The sun is the most damaging during the midday hours between 10 am and 2 pm. Being in the sun outside of those hours does not guarantee there will be no damage, but those times are generally considered the safest. A simple method for recognizing when to seek shade is called the shadow rule. The shorter your shadow, the greater your risk for sun damage. A person's shadow is shortest at midday, when the sun is highest in the sky.

Table 2-1. UV Index

UV Level	Category	Precautions
0 to 2	Low	Wear sunglasses with UV protection. Cover exposed skin with sunscreen SPF 30+ (if you easily burn).
3 to 5	Moderate	Wear sunglasses with UV protection. Wear a wide-brimmed hat and protective clothing. Cover exposed skin with sunscreen SPF 30+. Reapply every 2 hours.
6 to 7	High	Reduce your time in the sun between 10 am and 4 pm. Wear sunglasses with UV protection. Wear a wide-brimmed hat and protective clothing. Cover exposed skin with sunscreen SPF 30+. Reapply every 2 hours.
8 to 10	Very high	Minimize your time in the sun between 10 am and 4 pm. Wear sunglasses with UV protection. Wear a wide-brimmed hat and protective clothing. Cover exposed skin with sunscreen SPF 30+. Reapply every 2 hours.
11 or higher	Extreme	Avoid the sun between 10 am and 4 pm. Wear sunglasses with UV protection. Wear a wide-brimmed hat and protective clothing. Cover exposed skin with sunscreen SPF 30+. Reapply every 2 hours.

Note. Based on information from U.S. Environmental Protection Agency, n.d.-b.

The elevation of a specific location also factors into UV risk because the sun is farther away from places at sea level than places located at higher elevations. EPA also urges extra caution when around reflective surfaces like snow and water because the UV rays bounce back and deliver a second dose of UV at about 80% the original concentration.

Another major factor in UV exposure is season or time of year. Some U.S. locations, like Colorado, have very pronounced seasons, whereas Florida, for example, has very little seasonal diversity. This is one reason why using zip codes and seasonal information is helpful in predicting UV sun exposure.

Health Risks of Tanning Beds and Artificial UV Exposure

For most people, avoiding the sun altogether is unrealistic. However, purposefully exposing yourself to artificial UV radiation is completely avoidable—and should be. Indoor tanning beds and booths and sunlamps are an unsafe way to create a sun-bronzed look. Based on scientific evidence, the World Health Organization lists indoor tanning devices as carcinogenic (cancer causing) because of the increased risk for all three types of skin cancer: basal cell **carcinoma**, squamous cell carcinoma, and melanoma. Each of these types of cancer will be discussed later in this chapter.

Basic Skin and Eye Anatomy

The skin is the largest organ of the body and is made up of specialized cells distributed in three distinct layers (see Figure 2-1).

Figure 2-1. Skin Anatomy

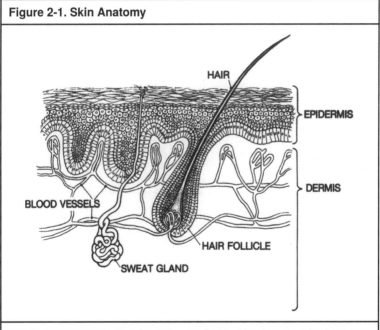

Note. Figure courtesy of National Cancer Institute. Retrieved from https://visualsonline.cancer.gov/details.cfm?imageid=1785.

The outermost and visible layer of the skin is called the *epidermis*. It houses immune cells and protects the body from foreign invaders and injury. The skin's middle and thickest layer is called the *dermis*. Along with storing water, the dermis controls body temperature. The **subcutaneous** layer is the deepest skin layer and contains mostly fat cells and connective tissue. This layer acts as a shock absorber and helps regulate body temperature.

Skin and eyelids contain specialized cells, including basal cells, squamous cells, **melanocytes**, and Merkel cells. Some are more likely than others to mutate and become cancerous.

Basal cells are found in the deepest part of the epidermis and produce new skin cells, which are pushed upward to the skin's surface. As basal cells mature and migrate to the skin's surface, they become squamous cells. Thicker than the parent basal cells, squamous cells produce a protective protein substance called *keratin*, which makes up hair and nails, so these cells are called *keratinocytes*.

Melanocytes produce *melanin*, the substance that gives the skin color. Melanin darkens skin tone in response to sun exposure; this is the body's way of protecting the skin from further damage. However, the deadliest form of skin cancer, melanoma, can occur when melanocytes are damaged and mutate.

FACT OR FICTION? African Americans do not get melanoma skin cancers.

Fiction. Darker skin produces more melanin, but it can still get sunburned and suffer UV damage leading to skin cancers, including melanoma. People with darker skin may have lower incidences of melanoma, but their skin cancers are often found at more advanced stages. People of all skin colors should wear sunscreen to avoid UV damage.

Merkel cells are responsible for the sensation of touch, and Merkel cell carcinoma is possible if these cells mutate. *Carcinoma* is the medical term for any cancer that develops in skin cells and cells on the outer or inner surface of organs like the lungs and liver.

Layers of the eyelid are different from those of the rest of the skin on the body, but many of the cellular components are the same. The eyelids are thin but do filter some UV rays. Over time, the structures of the eye that filter UV radiation and the eye itself can become damaged. According to the National Cancer Institute (NCI), the most common cancer of the eyelid is basal cell carcinoma, making up 90% of cases. Squamous cell carcinoma, melanoma, and other cancers make up the remaining 10% of eyelid cancers. Cancer of the eyelid can affect the eye itself, so prevention, early detection, and treatment can be lifesaving and reduce the loss of vision or the need for the removal of the eye. Cancer can also develop within the eye, although this is a rare occurrence, and immediate treatment is crucial.

Types of Cancerous Skin Lesions

Skin cancer is mostly preventable, yet when all types of skin cancer are grouped together, it is the most commonly diagnosed cancer in the United States. Overall, one in five Americans will experience at least one skin cancer diagnosis in their lifetime. Statistics on melanoma are most accurate because all cases of melanoma must be reported to the National Cancer Database Registry. Basal and squamous cell cancers, typically referred to as nonmelanoma skin cancer (NMSC), do not have to be reported, so data on these cancers are less precise. The American Cancer Society (ACS) estimates that 5.4 million cases of cancers starting in the basal and squamous cells are diagnosed each year. ACS expects melanoma to affect 87,110 people and cause nearly 9,730 deaths in 2017—an increase over previous years as the upward trend continues. Currently, melanoma is the fifth most common cancer in men and the sixth most common cancer in women. Melanoma is one of the most common cancers in adolescents and young adults and has risen with alarming frequency over the past 40 years.

For early detection and prevention purposes, any change in the color, shape, or size of a skin lesion (such as moles or sores) should be evaluated by your healthcare provider. Any new skin markings or a sore that is not healing may represent a cancerous condition and should also be evaluated. Nonmelanoma skin lesions are described in Figure 2-2.

Detection, Diagnosis, and Treatment of Nonmelanoma Skin Cancers

Detection, diagnosis, and treatment of NMSCs involves a skin examination and biopsy to remove some or all of the damaged tissue. Specialized physicians called **pathologists** examine the tissue under a microscope to look for malignant cells. Treatment for NMSC and actinic keratosis, a form of precancer, generally involves removal of the damaged cells by surgery, **cryotherapy** (freezing the tissue), or laser. Precisely delivered radiation therapy is another method used to kill cancer cells or keep them from growing. Several drugs can also be used to treat NMSC. Chemotherapy kills quickly dividing cells like skin cells. Biotherapies are medications that help the body recognize and kill cancer cells. Targeted therapies typically spare other body cells by attacking cancer cells directly. Photodynamic therapy uses both medications and a laser light to kill the cancer cells. Many of these same therapies are used to treat melanoma.

Melanoma

Recall that the melanocytes are part of the epidermis and are responsible for darkening the skin. Melanoma is a cancer of the melanocytes and is a much more aggressive cancer than both basal cell and squamous cell carcinomas; therefore, early detection and treatment are critical. Although melanoma is a relatively rare cancer, NCI reports that it accounts for 75% of deaths related to skin cancer. The incidence of melanoma is particularly rising in non-Hispanic Whites, men older than age 50, women younger than age 50, and older adults. Risk factors for melanoma include consistent sun exposure, fair skin that freckles or burns easily, family and personal history, multiple moles, and an inadequate immune system.

Figure 2-2. Nonmelanoma Skin Lesions

A. Actinic keratosis (precancerous lesion)
- May appear as a grouping of rough, raised, scaly skin cells appearing red, pink, or brown in color.
- When actinic keratosis develops on the lip, balm does not relieve the cracking and peeling.
- Associated with aging and can lead to squamous cell carcinoma.

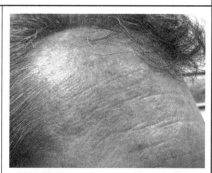

B. Basal cell carcinoma (cancer)
- 3 times more common than squamous cell carcinoma.
- May look like a flat patch of unusual skin or as a raised, pinkish-colored marking with a pearly rim or may appear as a sore, red patch, shiny bump, or scar.
- Rarely spreads to other parts of the body.

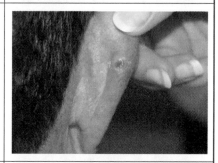

C. Squamous cell carcinoma (cancer)
- May look like a red, flat, scaly skin lesion, an open sore, or a bump with a crater in the center.
- Ears, scalp, face, neck, hands, and legs are particularly at risk for squamous cell cancers. Other susceptible areas include lips, eyelids, and genitals.
- People who use indoor tanning devices have a 2.5 times higher risk for developing squamous cell carcinoma.

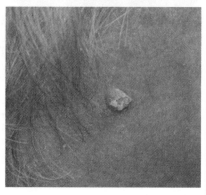

Note. Figure A courtesy of Future FarmDoc, 2014, licensed under Creative Commons Attribution-ShareAlike License (https://creativecommons.org/licenses/by-sa/4.0/deed.en). Retrieved from https://commons.wikimedia.org/wiki/File:Actinic_keratoses_on_forehead.JPG. Figures B and C courtesy of National Cancer Institute; Kelly Nelson, MD, photographer. Retrieved from https://visualsonline.cancer.gov/details.cfm?imageid=9235 and https://visuals online.cancer.gov/details.cfm?imageid=9248.

NCI widely encourages use of the ABCDE rule (see Figure 2-3), a simple method that can help identify changes in moles and other skin markings. Itching and bleeding of skin lesions are later signs of a potential melanoma. If you find any of these changes, talk with a dermatologist (a medical professional specializing in skin conditions).

Melanoma can spread into nearby tissue or to other parts of the body through the bloodstream or lymphatic system. **Lymph** nodes filter harmful substances from the body, so the nodes nearest to the melanoma lesion are also removed and examined for melanoma cells. Treatments and survival statistics are based on staging and national guidelines. The size and depth of the lesion, how

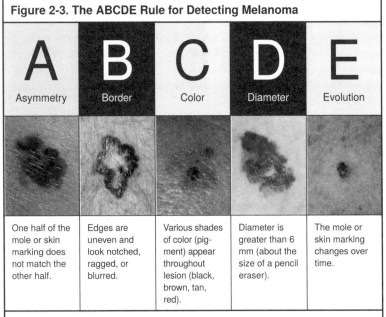

Figure 2-3. The ABCDE Rule for Detecting Melanoma

A	B	C	D	E
Asymmetry	Border	Color	Diameter	Evolution
One half of the mole or skin marking does not match the other half.	Edges are uneven and look notched, ragged, or blurred.	Various shades of color (pigment) appear throughout lesion (black, brown, tan, red).	Diameter is greater than 6 mm (about the size of a pencil eraser).	The mole or skin marking changes over time.

Note. Images courtesy of National Cancer Institute; Laurence Meyer, MD, PhD, University of Utah Health Sciences Center, photographer for images A, B, and D. Retrieved from https://visualsonline.cancer.gov/details.cfm?imageid=9244; https://visualsonline.cancer.gov/details.cfm?imageid=9245; https://visualsonline.cancer.gov/details.cfm?imageid=9291; https://visualsonline.cancer.gov/details.cfm?imageid=9247; and https://visualsonline.cancer.gov/details.cfm?imageid=9289.

quickly the melanoma cells are multiplying, and whether melanoma cells are found in the lymph nodes are used to determine melanoma stage and treatment. Immunotherapy, which helps the immune system recognize and destroy cancer cells, is currently the standard of care in melanoma treatment.

Skin Cancer Screening and Prevention

Skin cancer is a serious public health problem. The Centers for Disease Control and Prevention report more than $8 billion dollars are spent to treat skin cancer each year, and costs continue to rise. Skin cancer prevention is a high priority for national and local public health departments and is a major step toward reducing public health costs and, most importantly, increasing overall survival from a highly preventable cancer.

Skin Cancer Screening

The purpose of cancer screening is to find cancer before signs and symptoms are noticed. Mammograms and colonoscopies are common examples of screening studies. Agencies such as ACS, NCI, and the U.S. Preventive Services Task Force (USPSTF) make cancer screening recommendations based on evidence from clinical trials and other well-conducted studies. These agencies agree there is a lack of evidence showing better outcomes with routine skin cancer screening in the public. Therefore, there are no standard guidelines for how often a person should have a head-to-toe skin examination. People with a long history of sun exposure and sunburn are at risk for basal cell carcinoma, squamous cell carcinoma, and melanoma. Having a personal or family history of skin cancer, being fair-skinned, being age 65 years and older, and having more than 50 moles are considered risk factors for melanoma. USPSTF is reviewing studies examining how behavioral counseling may lead to improved sun protection behavior and performance of self-examinations.

Public health agencies encourage everyone to keep a watch on their own skin and have a healthcare provider look at suspicious lesions. Children should also be taught to watch for these skin changes. By using the ABCDE formula and documenting the location, color, and symptoms on a standard body map (see Figure 2-4), you can seek appropriate medical help.

Skin Cancer Prevention

Every skin type needs some degree of sun protection. The Fitzpatrick Skin Type Classification system (see Table 2-2) is one way of determining how much UV protection may be needed to prevent skin burning and damage, which could lead to skin cancer. Skin type is ranked on a scale of 1 (always burns, never tans, sensitive to UV exposure) to 6 (never burns, deeply pigmented, least sensitive). People with skin types 1 and 2 need more UV protection

Figure 2-4. Standard Body Map

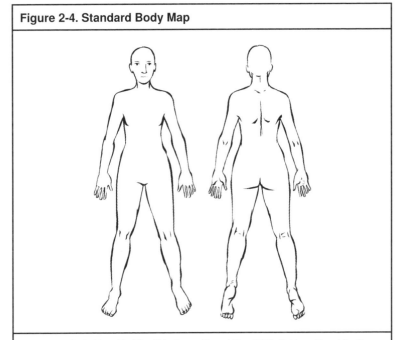

Note. From "Body Maps," by The Skin Cancer Foundation, 2016. Retrieved from http://www .skincancer.org/Media/Default/File/File/scf-body-map-2016.pdf. Copyright 2016 by The Skin Cancer Foundation. Reprinted with permission.

Table 2-2. Fitzpatrick Skin Type Classification	
Skin Type	**Reaction to Sun Exposure**
1	Always burns, never tans
2	Usually burns, tans minimally
3	Sometimes mildly burns, tans uniformly
4	Burns minimally, always tans well
5	Very rarely burns, tans very easily
6	Never burns, never tans

Note. Based on information from U.S. Department of Health and Human Services, 2015.

than people with naturally darker pigment. People with the lowest rates of melanoma include those with a higher Fitzpatrick Skin Type, such as those of African or Asian descent and Pacific Islanders. American Indians, Alaskan Natives, and Hispanic populations also have a lower incidence of melanoma than non-Hispanic Whites and people of European descent.

Applying sunscreen to exposed skin, wearing a hat and sunglasses with UV protection, and wearing UV-blocking clothes are strategies that can reduce the risk of skin cancer from naturally occurring UV radiation. Artificial sources of UV radiation, such as indoor tanning devices, can be even more damaging than natural UV light, especially for younger, frequent users. One sure way you can escape the risk of exposure to artificial UV radiation is to avoid all forms of unnatural exposure and follow the sun protection guidelines outlined in the 2015 *Surgeon General's Call to Action to Prevent Skin Cancer,* including sunscreen use and other measures.

Sunscreen Products

All sunscreen products are required to list a sun protection factor (SPF) and whether the product is considered broad spectrum, meaning it filters both UVA and UVB. The 2015 *Surgeon General's Call to Action to Prevent Skin Cancer* explains that a product with an SPF of 15 protects the skin 15 times longer than if the sunscreen was not used (SPF 30 protects 30 times longer, and so on). Using a sunscreen with SPF 15 blocks 93% of the sun's UV rays, SPF 30 blocks 97%, and SPF 50 blocks 98%. Broad-spectrum sunscreens SPF 15 or higher are recommended for adequate sun protection for most people. Products with an SPF lower than 15 and without broad-spectrum coverage may prevent sunburn but may not protect your skin from premature aging and damage. You should reapply sunscreen every two hours and more often if swimming or sweating. Using sunscreen properly has been shown to reduce the incidence of sunburn and skin cell damage. You are at risk for UV overexposure when you do not use sunscreen with an adequate SPF, apply sunscreen incorrectly, or use sunscreen as your only method of skin protection.

Consumers have listed cost, smell, mess, and inconvenience as barriers to proper sunscreen use. Concern that the ingredients in sunscreens may be unhealthy is another consumer issue; however, no large-scale human studies have been done to verify that the mineral or chemical components regularly used in sunscreens lead to skin cancer. In contrast, evidence shows that long-term UV damage can lead to skin cancer.

Some studies show that many Americans simply do not feel they are at high risk for skin cancer or do not fully understand how sunscreen and other sun protection methods can prevent signs of aging and skin cancer. Several government and private agencies are working to help better educate the public on sun protection and skin cancer prevention.

UV-Protective Clothing and Head Coverings

Some types of fabrics offer more UV protection than others. For example, hats and clothing made with tightly woven, light-colored fabrics offer more protection than similar products made from dark, loosely woven fabrics. Apparel incorporating extra UV protection is becoming more available, but the U.S. Food and Drug Administration does not regulate these claims of added protection, and the items typically cost more than items without added UV protection. Head coverings can be another important way to protect skin, but the fabric and design determine the level of protection. Large-brimmed hats offer the most protection for the face, neck, and shoulders. Hats with a loose weave, such as straw and other woven material, offer less protection.

UV-Protective Eyewear

The U.S. Food and Drug Administration cautions against judging sunglasses by their lens color. The amount of UV protection is not dependent on the darkness of the lens. A wraparound style with broad-spectrum 100% UV protection factor offers the best protection from direct and reflective UV exposure.

Special Considerations

Protection from UV overexposure is an important aspect of staying healthy overall. Using a combination of sun protection measures is recommended over using any one method alone. Additional care is needed for children, older adults, outdoor workers, and people with certain medical conditions.

Infants and Children

Skin damage earlier in life can cause cell mutations that may initially remain hidden but lead to cancer later in life. This is just one of the many reasons to start protecting infants and children from day one.

An infant's skin contains less melanin (skin pigment) and is more likely to sunburn. Infants' skin is also thinner and may be sensitive to sunscreen, so experts advise a simple solution: keep infants from birth to six months old out of direct sunlight. Cover infants' skin in clothing or coverings that block UV radiation. Remember, UVA and UVB can penetrate glass, so using a window shade or a UV-blocking film on windows can protect infants and children when riding in the car.

Severe sunburns in childhood increase the risk for melanoma and other skin cancers. This fact alone is reason to diligently protect children from UV radiation. Just like buckling up in the car, when adults model sun safety behaviors, children are more likely to make sun protection a lifelong habit. The sun safety methods discussed earlier in this chapter help protect children from UV radiation and the dangers of overexposure to UV radiation.

Older Adults

Sun protection for the older adult population is similar to protecting an infant's skin because of skin thinning and a less effective immune system with advancing age. Skin may also become more sensitive with age. Covering up with UV-protective clothing, using a sensitive-skin sunscreen on exposed areas such as the hands and back of the neck, and wearing wraparound sunglasses continue to be important protections for this population, as well.

Outdoor Workers

Overexposure to UV radiation is an occupational hazard for people who work outdoors. Remember, tanned skin may not burn as easily, but sun damage is still occurring. Ongoing, chronic exposure to UV radiation puts outdoor workers at a high risk for developing basal cell carcinoma and squamous cell carcinoma. Some studies suggest outdoor workers may be at less risk for melanoma, while other studies show an increased risk. There is agreement, however, that sun safety measures such as covering exposed skin, using SPF 15+ sunscreens, and wearing UV-protective eyewear are a must for people who work outside.

Medications and Medical Conditions

When taking some types of medications, people can become much more sensitive to UV radiation (a condition known as *photosensitivity*). For example, some antibiotics and chemotherapy drugs can cause a harmful effect by interacting with UV radiation and causing a rash-like burn, usually happening within 24 hours of sun exposure. Allergic reactions (itching, burning, redness, bumps) to topically applied products generally happen within a few days of sun exposure. Talk to a healthcare provider or pharmacist to understand the photosensitivity risks of specific medications.

An immune reaction to the sun can cause medical conditions such as lupus, polymorphous light eruption, and actinic prurigo, creating rash-like patches, bumps, and skin spots. Alternatively, other medical conditions can be treated with UV radiation, which is called *phototherapy*. Conditions such as psoriasis, actinic keratosis, and even basal cell carcinoma can be treated with combinations of medications and phototherapy, but these treatments are carefully supervised and use specific doses of UV radiation, which is very different than sun exposure, where the dose of radiation is dependent on other factors such as skin tone, UV index, and protection methods used.

Summary

Sun safety is important at any age. Overexposure to UV radiation can lead to sun damage, causing premature aging and skin cancer. Skin cancer is the most frequently diagnosed cancer in the United States, including basal cell carcinoma and squamous cell carcinoma. These cancers are less likely to spread beyond the skin. Melanoma, however, can easily spread to other areas and is one of the 10 most common cancers.

You can protect yourself from UVA and UVB radiation by covering exposed skin with clothing and wide-brimmed hats, applying sunscreen SPF 15+ before going out in the sun, or repeating sunscreen application every two hours (or more often if in the water or sweating). Other equally effective protections include wearing wraparound sunglasses with 100% UV protection, staying indoors or seeking shade during peak sun hours of 10 am to 2 pm, and avoiding artificial tanning devices. Sun safety doesn't have to be difficult. By remembering these strategies, your time in the sun can be safe and satisfying.

Recommended Reading

National Cancer Institute. (2016). Cancer statistics. Retrieved from https://www.cancer.gov/about-cancer/understanding/statistics

Shafie Pour, N., Saeedi, M., Morteza Semnani, K., & Akbari, J. (2015). Sun protection for children: A review. *Journal of Pediatrics Review, 3*, e155. doi:10.5812/jpr.155

Tripp, M.K., Watson, M., Balk, S.J., & Swetter, S.M. (2016). State of the science on prevention and screening to reduce melanoma incidence and mortality: The time is now. *CA: A Cancer Journal for Clinicians, 6,* 460–480. doi:10.3322/caac.21352

U.S. Department of Health and Human Services. (2015). *The Surgeon General's call to action to prevent skin cancer.* Retrieved from https://www.cdc.gov /cancer/skin/call_to_action/index.htm

Glossary

carcinoma [kahr-suh-noh-muh]—A cancerous and invasive epithelial tumor that spreads by metastasis and often recurs after excision.

cryotherapy [krahy-oh-ther-uh-pee]—Treatment by means of applications of cold.

dermis [dur-mis]—The dense inner layer of skin beneath the epidermis, composed of connective tissue, blood and lymph vessels, sweat glands, hair follicles, and an elaborate sensory nerve network.

epidermis [ep-i-dur-mis]—The outer, nonvascular, nonsensitive layer of the skin covering the true skin or dermis.

lymph [limf]—A clear yellowish, slightly alkaline, coagulable fluid containing white blood cells in a liquid resembling blood plasma derived from the tissues of the body and conveyed to the bloodstream by the lymphatic vessels.

melanocyte [meh-lan-oh-site]—A cell in the skin and eyes that produces and contains the pigment called melanin.

pathologist—A doctor who has special training in identifying diseases by studying cells and tissues under a microscope.

subcutaneous [sub-kyoo-tay-nee-us]—Beneath the skin.

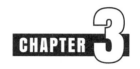

Screening for Cancer

Kristin Shea Donahue, RN, MSN, OCN®

> *Preventing or curing all cancers is our collective goal.*
> *We know today essentially how to prevent 100% of all*
> *deaths from cervical cancer. We are also able to prevent*
> *up to 30% of all deaths from breast cancer. This is not*
> *because of a new scientific breakthrough; it is because*
> *of cancer screening tests, some which have been around*
> *since the late 1940s.*
>
> —Otis Brawley, MD,
> American Cancer Society Chief Medical Officer,
> Statement to the Committee on Oversight
> and Government Reform,
> U.S. House of Representatives, January 29, 2008

Although the prevention of cancer is surely everyone's goal, a cancer diagnosis is sometimes unavoidable. Early detection is key to giving those diagnosed the best chance of a successful outcome. Finding cancer at a later stage may limit treatment options. Screening tools have led to earlier detection of cancer, thus saving lives. Unfortunately, not all cancers have screening options available. Researchers are working to improve current screening tools and develop even more options so we can detect more cancers earlier.

Screening refers to tests and examinations done on people who are not showing any symptoms associated with cancer. Once people have symptoms, such as pain, functional changes, or noticeable changes in health, healthcare providers use diagnostic tools rather than screening tools to diagnose cancer. Screenings can include a physical examination, blood tests, imaging studies, and genetic testing. Chapter 10 discusses genetic testing in further detail, so it will not be discussed as a screening option in this chapter.

It is important to talk with your healthcare provider about your health history and family history to decide what cancer screening tools are right for you. Screening tools play an important role in diagnosing cancer early; however, they can have risks. Although it is rare, some tests can cause injury when performed. Your provider should explain these risks before you have any screening done so you can decide if the benefits outweigh the risks.

The potential for a false-positive or a false-negative test result is an area of concern associated with cancer screenings. A *false-positive* result occurs when a screening tool incorrectly suggests a person has cancer. This type of result can cause needless worry to a person and can lead to further unnecessary tests and associated costs. A *false-negative* result occurs when the screening tool incorrectly suggests a person does not have cancer, but in fact, the person does. This kind of result can lead to delays in care and a false sense of security.

The overdiagnosis of cancer is another risk factor related to cancer screening. Although this may not seem like a bad thing, many types of cancer go undetected for many years without causing any issues, and individuals can outlive their cancers. In other words, it could do more harm than good for a person to know he or she had cancer. For example, a woman in her mid-80s may die of natural causes before her nonmelanoma skin cancer causes any issues. Would it be best to let her live out her days without the stress and anxiety of knowing she has cancer? Would she have to undergo unnecessary treatments that may decrease her quality of life yet not prolong her life at all? These can be difficult questions to answer, and certainly, every situation is different.

This chapter discusses the most common types of cancer and the available cancer screening tools. Research and development of screening tools is ongoing for many different types of cancer, so although a specific cancer may not have a screening tool available today, one may exist in the future.

The screening tools and guidelines discussed here are meant for people who have an average risk of developing cancer. People with a genetic risk or family history of cancer may have different screening criteria. Not all screenings discussed here are recommended by every healthcare organization. It is important to discuss your risks with your healthcare team to determine the tests that are most appropriate for you. Please use this information as a general guide when considering screening tools.

Screening Tools by Cancer Type

Colon Cancer

Many screening tools are available for colon cancer, which is great news considering colorectal cancer is the second leading cause of cancer deaths. Options range from highly invasive procedures done in medical facilities to much less invasive tests done at home. There are differing opinions on what tests should be done and how often. The three most widely accepted tests for colon cancer screening are colonoscopy, sigmoidoscopy, and fecal occult blood test (FOBT). All tests have benefits and risks, so discussing these risks with healthcare providers is essential.

Colonoscopy

A colonoscopy is the gold-standard procedure used to screen for colon cancer. People at average risk for colon cancer should have a colonoscopy starting at age 50 and every 10 years thereafter. During the procedure, the provider places a colonoscope—a type of endoscope, or a long, flexible camera—through the rectum and into the colon. The entire colon is viewed during a colonoscopy. The provider may also perform a biopsy, which is the collection of a tissue sample, during the colonoscopy if abnormalities are present. Generally, patients have little to no side effects related to the colonoscopy; however, the procedure requires sedation. People tolerate sedation differently, so experiences may vary.

A slight risk of bleeding or bowel **perforation** is associated with a colonoscopy. Although this complication is rare, it is something to consider when preparing for a colonoscopy. Because the entire colon is visualized during a colonoscopy, the entire colon must be cleared. Bowel preparation will vary based on each healthcare facility, but it generally includes a clear liquid diet the day before the colonoscopy. A laxative, typically in the form of a drink, will also be given the day before the procedure. It is important to drink plenty of fluids the day before the procedure to help flush out the colon. Another laxative may be recommended the day of the procedure a few hours in advance to ensure the bowel is completely clear. No food of any kind is allowed the day of the procedure until after it is complete.

During the procedure, the provider will pump air into the colon to ensure proper visibility. This can cause cramping and bloating. Advantages to the colonoscopy are that it visualizes the entire colon and is only necessary every 10 years for those at average risk for colon cancer.

Flexible Sigmoidoscopy

People at average risk for colon cancer should consider having a sigmoidoscopy starting at age 50 and every five years thereafter. During the procedure, a sigmoidoscope, another type of endoscope, is passed through the rectum and into the **sigmoid colon**, which is the lower portion of the colon. If any abnormalities, such as **polyps**, are found during the procedure, a healthcare provider will biopsy the polyps at the same time. Although there is always a chance that the bowel can be punctured during the procedure, patients typically tolerate the procedure well and usually do not require sedation. The lower colon must be cleared of stool prior to the procedure, so some colon preparation is required, but this is typically less comprehensive than a colonoscopy bowel preparation. As with a colonoscopy, patients can experience bloating and cramping because of the air pumped into the colon; however, both usually stop shortly after the procedure.

High-Sensitivity Fecal Occult Blood Tests

High-sensitivity FOBTs detect blood in the stool and have a high accuracy rate in detecting cancer. Some polyps and colon cancer can cause bleeding, so this test can be effective in detecting them. Although blood in the stool does not necessarily mean that a person has polyps or colon cancer, it is something that should be investigated further. Patients can collect a sample at home and return it to their healthcare providers to complete the test. How often patients should be tested is still up for debate. However, it is widely accepted and recommended that the average-risk person should begin having FOBTs at age 50 and should continue until age 80. The U.S. Preventive Services Task Force recommends FOBT be performed every year if it is the only test being used to screen for colon cancer. Currently, two types of high-sensitivity FOBTs—gFOBT and iFOBT—are approved by the U.S. Food and Drug Administration.

The guaiac fecal occult blood test (gFOBT) can be performed at home. Individuals use a kit to collect one or more samples of stool. Once the sample is collected, individuals return the kit back to the healthcare provider to complete the test. The gFOBT screens for blood in the stool by using a chemical to detect heme, a component of hemoglobin found in red blood cells. Screening for blood in the stool is important because both polyps and colon cancer can cause bleeding. However, not all precancerous or cancerous polyps bleed, in which case, the gFOBT would not detect any abnormalities. Specific foods, such as red meats and certain vegetables, should be avoided prior to having a gFOBT because they can cause a false-positive result. Individuals completing a gFOBT should also tell their providers about all medications they are taking, including vitamins, as these can alter the test results.

Unlike the gFOBT, the fecal immunochemical test (FIT or iFOBT) uses antibodies to test for human hemoglobin in the stool and thus determine if blood is present in the stool. Unlike the gFOBT, dietary restrictions are usually not required for the FIT. It should also be performed annually if used as the only colon cancer screening method.

Single-Specimen Guaiac Fecal Occult Blood Test

The single-specimen gFOBT is different from high-sensitivity FOBTs in that this test is performed in a medical facility by a healthcare provider. The stool sample is typically collected during a digital rectal examination when a healthcare provider inserts a finger into the rectum. This is not a recommended screening for colon cancer because it is considered outdated.

Stool DNA Test

The stool DNA test (sDNA test or FIT-DNA test) can also be done at home. Individuals receive a kit to collect and mail an entire stool sample. The test not only looks for blood in the stool but also tests for nine DNA biomarkers. These specific biomarkers can be found in genes linked to precancerous and cancerous colon lesions that slough off and remain in the stool. If an individual's sample tests positive for blood or the DNA biomarkers, a colonoscopy is recommended. Even though many organizations state the sDNA test should be done every one to three years, there are currently no consistent recommendations on the frequency of this test. Health insurance may not cover this test.

Virtual Colonoscopy

A virtual colonoscopy, also known as a computed tomography (CT) colonography, uses a CT scan to take pictures of the inside of the colon and rectum. The procedure is less invasive because no equipment is inserted into the body. It also does not require any sedation like the standard colonoscopy. A virtual colonoscopy still requires colon preparation to clear the bowel to get the best possible images. Cramping and bloating are common side effects because the procedure requires air to be pumped into the colon. The virtual colonoscopy has similar accuracy as that of the colonoscopy. If an abnormality such as a polyp is discovered, a standard colonoscopy must be performed. Still, for those who are not interested in a more invasive procedure such as the colonoscopy, this may be a good screening option. However, many insurance companies do not cover the cost of a virtual colonoscopy. People considering having a virtual colonoscopy should check with their health insurance companies prior to having the procedure to find out what insurance will cover and if they will have any out-of-pocket costs.

Camera Pill

The camera pill takes photographs inside the colon. Individuals swallow the pill following bowel preparation, and the pill can take up to 10 hours to move through the colon. Patients need to limit their activity to ensure the camera moves through the colon in the appropriate amount of time. The camera will leave the body through a bowel movement and does not need to be retrieved because it transmits images to a wearable device. Currently, only individuals who are not able to complete a colonoscopy are given this option for screening.

Double-Contrast Barium Enema

A double-contrast barium enema combines the use of an x-ray and a barium solution to take images of the inside of the colon and rectum to monitor for any abnormalities. Prior to the x-ray, a barium solution is delivered into the patient's rectum and colon. This solution helps to provide a better picture of the colon by outlining the anatomy of the colon and rectum. Double-contrast barium enema is not recommended as the standard screening tool for colon cancer because it is less accurate in detecting abnormalities such as polyps. This procedure may still be recommended for individuals who are unable to undergo a colonoscopy.

Advances in Colon Cancer Screening

Researchers are working to develop new, less invasive tests to detect colon cancer. They are also looking at other biomarker tests that could help to detect colon cancer at its earliest stage. Your healthcare providers can help you determine which tests are appropriate. People with a personal or family history of polyps or colon cancer may need more frequent screenings.

Breast Cancer

Although it largely affects women, breast cancer can develop in both women and men, as men also have breast tissue. Currently, medical professionals use several screening tools to detect breast cancer, the most common being the mammogram. Other commonly used screening options include breast ultrasound, magnetic resonance imaging (MRI) scans, breast self-examinations, and clinical breast examinations. If you have a family history of breast cancer, it is important to talk with a healthcare provider to decide the best screening tools. Genetic testing may also be an option in screening for breast cancer. Please see Chapter 10 for more details about genetic testing for breast cancer.

Mammography

A mammogram is an x-ray of the breasts and is considered the standard of care in breast cancer screening. Each breast is placed on the surface of the mammogram machine and compressed to get a clear picture. The machine produces a picture of the inside of the breast, which the healthcare team examines for abnormalities, such as tumors. Although mammograms are considered safe, there are some things to consider before having one. Mammograms are a reliable way to detect breast cancer, but they are not perfect. They may not always show cancer when, in fact, it is present—a false-negative result. Mammograms may also show tumors that, once biopsied, prove to be harmless. Mammograms also expose those undergoing the test to radiation. However, the amount of radiation from a mammogram is typically smaller than that of a chest x-ray and is considered safe.

Although the mammogram is widely accepted as the preferred method for breast cancer screening, opinions differ on when women should start having mammograms and for how long they should continue to be screened. According to the American Cancer Society (ACS), women with an average risk for breast cancer may begin having mammograms between the ages of 40 and 44 and should definitely begin yearly mammograms by age 45. Based on ACS recommendations, women should continue to have yearly mammograms until age 55. At that time, women may choose to have mammograms every other year. ACS recommends that women continue mammogram screening until their life expectancy is less than 10 years. Women should talk with their healthcare provider to determine the best screening schedule.

Tomosynthesis

Tomosynthesis is a newer kind of digital mammography and is becoming more common in healthcare settings across the United States. It produces a three-dimensional view of the breast rather than the two-dimensional view of traditional mammography.

Breast Ultrasound

An ultrasound uses sound waves to see breast tissues. It may be used to examine lumps that cannot be easily seen by mammography. A breast ultrasound is also used to see the differences in lumps that can be fluid-filled cysts or solid masses, which a healthcare provider will treat differently.

Clinical Breast Examinations

A healthcare provider performs clinical breast examinations. The provider palpates, or touches, the breasts, feeling and looking for any abnormal changes. Opinions differ about the usefulness of performing clinical breast examinations because providers can also produce both false-negative and false-positive results, and having clinical breast examinations has not proven to reduce a person's risk of dying from breast cancer. Presently, it is still common for a healthcare provider to examine breasts during yearly physicals or wellness examinations.

Breast Self-Examinations

A breast self-examination is performed when an individual looks and feels for changes in her or his breasts. The examination is performed by feeling around the breast in a circular motion for any changes such as lumps or thickening of the breast tissue. The nipples and armpits should also be examined for changes.

Although the effectiveness of performing breast self-examinations is up for debate, with many organizations agreeing they have not reduced the risk of dying from breast cancer, a woman should know her body and identify any changes that may have occurred.

Magnetic Resonance Imaging

Although an MRI is not typically used to screen for breast cancer, it may be used in addition to mammography in people who are at increased risk for breast cancer. Those at an increased risk include individuals who have a genetic mutation or a first-degree relative with a genetic mutation, such as the *BRCA* mutation, Li-Fraumeni syndrome, Cowden syndrome, or Bannayan-Riley-Ruvalcaba syndrome. Other groups at increased risk include those who have had radiation exposure to the chest between the ages of 10 and 30 and individuals who have a 20%–25% increased risk for breast cancer compared to the general population. Providers calculate this percentage based on family history and personal medical history.

When an MRI is performed, IV contrast may be given before or during the test to aid in developing a clear, detailed image of the breast tissue. The IV contrast is a liquid that is injected into a vein and helps to make the area of the body being imaged stand out from other areas for a better picture.

Ovarian Cancer

Ovarian cancer is the fifth leading cause of cancer death in women in the United States. It is so deadly because many times it is not diagnosed until its later stages. Symptoms are often unclear and can be similar to other illnesses, making it difficult to diagnose. Currently, for those at average risk for ovarian cancer, no screening tools are approved. For those at *increased* risk for ovarian cancer, the effectiveness of other screenings, such as cancer **antigen** 125 (CA-125) testing and transvaginal ultrasound, is still up for debate.

Cancer Antigen 125 Tumor Marker

CA-125 is a naturally occurring protein in the body and can be measured by a blood test. It is called a *tumor marker* because it is usually elevated in women with ovarian cancer. However, it can also be elevated in women who do not have cancer, so it is not recommended as an ovarian cancer screening tool for women of average risk.

Transvaginal Ultrasound

During a transvaginal ultrasound, a healthcare provider inserts a probe into the vagina to examine the ovaries. The ultrasound uses sound waves to produce images and can show abnormalities. Further tests may be required if the test reveals irregularities. A transvaginal ultrasound is not a recommended ovarian cancer screening tool for women of average risk.

Women at high risk for ovarian cancer, such as those with a genetic mutation, should meet with healthcare providers, including a genetic counselor, to determine appropriate ongoing tests and care.

Prostate Cancer

Prostate cancer is the leading type of cancer in men, with one in seven men diagnosed in his lifetime. Widespread disagreement between healthcare organizations has led to no single standardized prostate cancer screening. The prostate-specific antigen (PSA) test was once considered the gold standard for prostate screening. Doctors no longer recommend it as the sole prostate cancer screening tool, and it is being researched more for use in the general population.

Currently, ACS recommends that men at average risk for prostate cancer discuss screening options with healthcare providers starting at age 50 if they are expected to live at least 10 years following the test. This may seem unusual, but prostate cancer typically grows slowly, and individuals can live for many years with the disease. It is important for men to talk with their healthcare providers and share in the decision making for prostate cancer screening options and frequency.

For men at high risk for prostate cancer, ACS recommends screening beginning at age 45. High-risk men include those who have first-degree relatives (father, brother, or son) diagnosed with prostate cancer and African Americans.

Researchers continue to look for ways to improve current prostate cancer screening options and develop better screening tools to help detect prostate cancer early. As always, it is important for men to talk with their healthcare providers to determine what tools and frequencies are best.

Prostate-Specific Antigen Test

This test detects the level of PSA, a protein produced by the prostate, in the blood. PSA is normally found in the blood, but increased levels may indicate prostate cancer. A healthcare provider may conduct a prostate biopsy in the case of increased PSA levels. Although most men with prostate cancer have an elevated PSA, this is not always the case, which can lead to false-negative tests. False-positive PSA tests can occur for other reasons, such as inflammation, infections, and medications. A single test may not be enough to diagnose prostate cancer. Having serial, or repeated, PSA tests may be a better indicator in diagnosing prostate cancer because a rising PSA can be tracked over time. Remember, screening and diagnosing prostate cancer are very different, and as mentioned, the PSA test is not a recommended prostate cancer screening tool by itself.

Digital Rectal Examination

A healthcare professional will often perform a digital rectal examination to check both the rectum and the prostate during a man's annual wellness checkup. During the examination, the provider inserts a lubricated finger into the rectum to feel for any abnormalities within the rectum or on the prostate. Digital rectal examination is not a recommended prostate cancer screening tool by itself. However, it is often used in combination with the PSA test as an appropriate prostate cancer screening option for some men. Healthcare providers will conduct further testing if they find any abnormalities.

Watchful Waiting

Based on individual risk factors, some healthcare professionals may choose to perform less testing while maintaining appointments to monitor potential prostate cancer growth. Many health-care professionals prefer not to use the term *watchful waiting*, as it can imply that nothing is happening in care; however, this is not the case. They may be providing the least invasive care to see if any symptoms develop. This is a reasonable approach for slow-growing cancers such as prostate cancer.

Cervical Cancer

Screening for cervical cancer has been one of the biggest suc-cess stories in the fight against cancer. The Pap test has helped drastically reduce the number of cervical cancer deaths over the past 30 years in the United States. ACS data indicate screen-ings have led to more than a 50% reduction in the number of cervical cancer deaths. Today, most cervical cancer cases occur in women who have never had a cervical screening or have not been screened in several years. Although the number of deaths from cervical cancer has dropped steeply in the United States, cervical cancer deaths around the world are still high because of the lack of access to screening. The Pap test is the standard test used to screen for cervical cancer, but human papillomavirus (HPV) testing may also be done in combination with Pap test-ing. This virus can cause cell changes that lead to cervical can-cer. Women who have had the HPV vaccination (discussed in more detail in Chapter 7) should continue to be screened for cervical cancer. Women should discuss their personal health his-tory with their healthcare providers to determine which tests to do and how often.

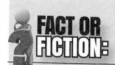 **FACT OR FICTION: Women who have had a hysterectomy no longer need cervical cancer screening.**

Fact. Women who have had a complete hysterectomy no longer need to have cervical screening. However, women who have had a supracervi-cal hysterectomy, meaning that their cervix is still intact, should continue to have cervical screenings.

Papanicolaou Test

A healthcare professional performs the Pap test, or Pap smear as it is often called, during a pelvic examination, and it is the standard screening for cervical cancer. This test samples cells from the cervix to determine if any abnormalities are present. The cervix is the narrow area that connects the uterus and vagina. A small instrument such as a brush or swab is inserted into the vagina and used to scrape cells from the **exocervix**, which is the outer area of the cervix. Another swab or brush is then used to collect cells from the **endocervix**, or inside of the cervix. The cell samples are sent to a lab where a healthcare provider uses a microscope to look for cancer or any precancerous changes. If an abnormality is found, several different options are available based on the results. They can range from continual monitoring with a Pap test to biopsies and surgical procedures.

Women should begin Pap screening at age 21. Currently, several organizations, including ACS and the American College of Obstetricians and Gynecologists, agree that a Pap test every three years is appropriate for the general population. Women may need more frequent screening if they have a history of an abnormal Pap test. Pap screening after age 65 is no longer recommended for women who have had three negative screening tests within the previous 10 years.

FACT OR FICTION: Cancer screenings should stop at certain ages.

Fact. Just as cancer screenings begin at certain ages, all currently recommended cancer screenings also stop at certain ages because the risks of the screening outweigh the benefits. Recommendations can change based on personal or family history, as well as current health and functional status.

Human Papillomavirus Cotest

An HPV cotest is a combination of the Pap test and HPV DNA testing, which detects the presence of HPV. The test uses the same cell samples scraped from in and around the cervix to test for HPV, so no additional samples are needed. Women aged 30 and older should have the test done every five years. Testing may stop after age 65.

High-Risk Human Papillomavirus Testing

The National Cancer Institute indicates high-risk HPV, or hrHPV, testing detects 14 different strains of HPV, which account for approximately 70% of cervical cancers. The collection method is the same as during a Pap test. It can be done with or without a Pap test, but healthcare organizations do not yet recommend hrHPV testing alone.

Lung Cancer

Lung cancer is the leading cause of cancer death in the United States for both men and women. More people die of lung cancer each year than colon, breast, and prostate cancers combined. Although lung cancer can be associated with a poor **prognosis** or outcome, people diagnosed with lung cancer at an early stage have quite a good prognosis. According to the National Cancer Institute, early detection of lung cancer can increase survival rates by 20%. Three tests have been studied to determine if they are effective lung screenings: chest x-ray, CT scan, and sputum cytology. A chest x-ray does not provide a good picture of the lungs for diagnosing lung cancer. It often misses nodules in the lungs, so it is not recommended as a good screening tool. Studies have determined that sputum cytology is also ineffective in screening for lung cancer. Presently, a low-dose CT scan is the only effective tool for early detection of lung cancer.

During a low-dose CT scan, medical professionals use a CT scanner to take multiple images of the lungs. The pictures are more detailed than an average x-ray, as the CT scan uses multiple pictures of small sections of the body to create one detailed picture. The scan does not require any oral or IV contrast and typically only takes about five minutes to perform.

Although the test is considered safe, there are risks. The scan does give off a small amount of radiation. The radiation exposure is minimal, but a healthcare provider should explain the risks prior to the test. A low-dose CT detects nodules, which may be either cancerous or noncancerous. Further testing and biopsies may be needed if the scan reveals nodules.

Although healthcare professionals recommend a low-dose CT scan for lung cancer screening, it is not for everyone. Individuals must meet certain criteria: must be a current or previous smoker (who has quit within the past 15 years), be 55–80 years old, and have at least a 30-pack-year smoking history. To determine a pack-year, multiply the number of packs smoked per day by the number of years smoked. For example, if a man smoked one pack of cigarettes each day for 45 years, his pack-year history would be 45. Individuals aged 50–54 who have at least a 20-pack-year smoking history and one other risk factor, such as environmental carcinogen exposure (radon or asbestos), family history of lung cancer, chronic lung disease, or a personal history of lung cancer, may also be candidates for lung screening. Currently, individuals who meet these criteria should have yearly lung screenings. If an individual has three consecutive negative lung screenings, a doctor may recommend stopping the screening. However, if the individual still smokes, the healthcare provider may determine that it is appropriate to have annual lung screenings. People who meet the criteria but are also experiencing symptoms, such as blood in the sputum, no longer qualify for low-dose CT screening. Instead, they will undergo diagnostic tests to determine potential causes of the symptoms.

Many individuals will have abnormal lung screenings without having lung cancer. Finding a nodule with low-dose CT does not necessarily mean a person will be diagnosed with lung cancer. Based on the size and number of lung nodules, the healthcare provider will determine a follow-up plan. Often, providers will do serial lung screenings over several months to determine if the nodule or nodules are growing or are stable and likely not cancerous.

Current or former smokers should talk with their healthcare providers to determine if low-dose CT lung cancer screening is appropriate.

Adrenal Cancer

Currently, no approved cancer screening tests exist for those at average risk for adrenal cancer. People with an inherited disorder such as Li-Fraumeni syndrome, Beckwith-Wiedemann syndrome, or Carney complex should be closely monitored by their healthcare providers, as they may have an increased risk of adrenal cancer.

Anal Cancer

Although the medical community has not agreed on a screening tool for anal cancer, men older than age 50 should have a rectal examination performed during their annual physical. Women who are sexually active should also have a rectal examination when they have their annual pelvic examination. Individuals at increased risk for anal cancer include men who have had sex with other men, individuals who are HIV positive, women who have had cervical or vulvar cancer, or anyone who has had an organ transplant. These people should talk with their healthcare providers about having further testing to screen for anal cancer.

Although the exact cause of anal cancer is not known, research indicates a link exists between HPV and anal cancer. Just as the Pap test has been used to help identify cervical cancer, the anal Pap test may be beneficial in identifying anal cancer.

The anal Pap test comprises inserting a swab into the rectum and collecting cells. The cells are then examined under a microscope to determine if any abnormalities exist. If an abnormality is found, providers may need to perform further testing and treatment. Currently, no set screening criteria exist for how often the test should be performed. Some literature suggests anal Pap testing every year for men who are HIV positive and every two to three years for men who do not have HIV. There are also no current recommendations for anal Pap testing in women, but women should talk with their healthcare providers regarding their risk for anal cancer to decide the best plan of care.

Bladder Cancer

For people with an average risk of bladder cancer, there are no established bladder cancer screening tests. However, healthcare providers may use a **hematuria** test, which identifies blood in the urine, along with other diagnostic tools to assist in identifying bladder cancer when symptoms exist.

Hematuria Test

A hematuria test determines if blood is present in the urine. Although this test can be used to help diagnose bladder cancer, having blood in the urine does not necessarily mean that an individual has bladder cancer. Many other disorders can cause blood in the urine; providers will perform further testing to discover the cause of blood in the urine.

Cystoscopy and Urine Cytology

Two tests—cystoscopy and urine cytology—are used to screen patients who have previously had bladder cancer. A healthcare provider decides how often to do these tests.

During a cystoscopy, a small, thin tube with a camera called a *cystoscope* is inserted into the bladder to examine it and look for irregularities. If abnormalities are found, a biopsy may be done at the time of the cystoscopy.

Urine cytology, a laboratory test, is used to examine a person's urine. A healthcare provider views the cells in the urine under a microscope to look for abnormalities. Further testing may be needed if any abnormalities are present.

Endometrial Cancer

Cancer of the endometrium (the mucous membrane lining of the uterus) is typically diagnosed at an early stage, thus giving the disease a high cure rate. Doctors can detect endometrial cancer early because it usually presents with symptoms such as abnormal bleeding. Remember, screening tests detect cancer when no symptoms are present. Currently, the healthcare community has no recommendations on standard screening tests for women at average risk for endometrial cancer. Individuals who have **Lynch syndrome** or a family history of Lynch syndrome, which is also known as *hereditary nonpolyposis colon cancer* (or HNPCC), are at an increased risk for endometrial cancer and should discuss high-risk screening options with their healthcare providers.

Kidney Cancer

For those at average risk for kidney cancer, no approved screenings are currently available. Individuals with an increased risk of developing kidney cancer need to be followed closely by their medical teams. Those at increased risk include people with a family history of kidney cancer and people with a genetic disorder. For high-risk individuals, such as those with von Hippel-Lindau disease, a healthcare team should closely monitor their cases. They may also need regular imaging screenings, which may include CT scans, MRIs, and ultrasounds.

Retinoblastoma

Retinoblastoma is a cancer of the eye, specifically the **retina** or rear part of the eye. Children younger than age three are most commonly diagnosed with this cancer. Currently, the American Academy of Pediatrics recommends a red reflex eye examination for newborns before being discharged from the hospital and on all routine health visits.

A healthcare provider conducts a red reflex examination by using an ophthalmoscope to shine a light into both eyes at the same time in a darkened room. The healthcare provider looks for a red reflection from both eyes, which is normal as light bounces off the retina. An abnormal finding can include a different response from one eye to the other, a white reflection, or dark spots. Typically, a white reflection will appear with retinoblastomas, and if this response occurs, the healthcare provider may refer the child to an ophthalmologist for further testing.

Skin Cancer

According to the National Cancer Institute, one in five people in the United States will be diagnosed with skin cancer at some point in their life, making it the most common type of cancer in the United States. As discussed in Chapter 2, several different types of skin cancer exist, but the deadliest is melanoma. All types of skin cancer have a high cure rate when detected early. The American Academy of Dermatology recommends skin self-examinations and yearly examinations by dermatologists to screen for skin cancer. These skin checks can detect skin cancer early and allow for more favorable outcomes.

Everyone should be aware of skin changes, including changes in the color, shape, and feel of moles or spots on the skin, and report any changes to a healthcare provider. A dermatologist can perform a yearly skin check in the office, often a full-body skin check, where the healthcare professional will view all areas of the patient's body for any skin changes. Although a yearly skin check is the recommendation for most people, a healthcare provider may determine that more frequent skin checks are necessary. Discussing skin cancer risk factors with a healthcare provider helps patients determine the best screening schedule.

Testicular Cancer

No screening tests are currently approved for those at average risk for testicular cancer. Although research has not shown testicular self-examinations to be effective as a screening tool, it is important for men to know their bodies to recognize any changes.

Thyroid Cancer

Currently, no medical tests are approved to screen for thyroid cancer in people at average risk. During annual wellness examinations, healthcare providers examine the neck to check for nodules or enlargement of the thyroid. If any abnormalities exist, the provider may do additional testing.

Other Cancers

Currently, no approved screenings are available for people with an average risk of developing the following cancers:

- Brain
- Esophageal
- Gastrointestinal stromal tumors
- Leukemia
- Lymphoma
- Multiple myeloma (cancer of blood plasma cells)
- Osteosarcoma (bone)
- Pancreatic

Summary

People need to openly discuss their health and family histories with their healthcare providers to determine the most appropriate cancer screening tools and frequencies. Screening tools are not without risks, so it is important to consider the risks and benefits and discuss those with healthcare providers to make an informed decision. Ultimately, preventing cancer is the goal, but early detection of cancer can improve outcomes and save lives. Most cancers have very favorable outcomes when diagnosed early, so everyone should be diligent in completing cancer screenings.

New screening tools are rapidly being developed to help detect cancer at its earliest stages. Although every effort was made to include all current screening tools in this chapter, it is possible that new screening tools have been developed since this book was published. It is also possible that screening guidelines may have changed because of new research and evidence. To understand the most up-to-date cancer screening guidelines, talk with your healthcare provider.

Recommended Reading

American Cancer Society. (2015). American Cancer Society guidelines for the early detection of cancer. Retrieved from http://www.cancer.org/healthy /findcancerearly/cancerscreeningguidelines/american-cancer-society -guidelines-for-the-early-detection-of-cancer

National Cancer Institute. (2016). Cancer screening overview (PDQ®) [Patient version]. Retrieved from http://www.cancer.gov/about-cancer /screening/patient-screening-overview-pdq

U.S. Preventive Services Task Force. (2015). Lung cancer: Screening. Retrieved from http://www.uspreventiveservicestaskforce.org/Page/ Document/UpdateSummaryFinal/lung-cancer-screening

Glossary

antigen [an-ti-jen]—1. Immunology: any substance that can stimulate the production of antibodies and combine specifically with them; 2. Pharmacology: any commercial substance that, when injected or absorbed into animal tissues, stimulates the production of antibodies.

endocervix—The mucous membrane of the uterine cervical canal.

exocervix—The portion of the uterine cervix extending into the vagina and lined with stratified squamous epithelium.

hematuria [hee-muh-too-ree-uh]—The presence of blood in the urine.

heme [heem]—A deep-red, iron-containing blood pigment obtained from hemoglobin.

Lynch syndrome—An inherited disorder in which affected individuals have a higher than normal chance of developing colorectal cancer and certain other types of cancer, often before the age of 50. Also called hereditary nonpolyposis colon cancer (HNPCC).

perforation—A rupture in a body part caused especially by accident or disease.

polyp [pah-lip]—A growth that protrudes from a mucous membrane.

prognosis [prog-no-sis]—The likely outcome or course of a disease; the chance of recovery or recurrence.

retina [reh-tih-nuh]—The light-sensitive layers of nerve tissue at the back of the eye that receive images and send them as electric signals through the optic nerve to the brain.

serial—Occurring in a series rather than simultaneously.

sigmoid colon—The S-shaped section of the colon that connects to the rectum.

CHAPTER 4

Physical Activity

Katrina Fetter, MSN, RN, AOCNS®, AGCNS-BC

> *If we could give every individual the right amount
> of nourishment and exercise, not too little and not
> too much, we would have found the safest way to
> health.*
>
> —Hippocrates

Nearly all of us are physically active at some point in our lives. *Physical activity* is defined as any movement from the muscles that needs more energy than resting. Four main types of physical activity exist:

- Aerobic—to strengthen the heart and lungs; commonly known as cardio
- Strengthening—to keep muscles, bones, and joints strong
- Flexibility and stretching—to help with everyday tasks and prepare the body for more strenuous exercise
- Balance—to maintain posture and prevent falls

People tend to be more physically active in their youth, but it is important to stay active as we get older. Staying active has many benefits, such as controlling weight and lowering the chances of heart disease, type 2 diabetes, high blood pressure, and stroke. Exercise also builds and maintains strong bones and muscles, along with keeping a pleasant mood. Regular activity raises the chances of living longer and prevents certain types of cancer.

FACT OR FICTION: Only healthy people can do physical activity.

Fiction. People can be active at almost any age whether they are "healthy" or not. With a provider's okay, even people with acute or long-term health issues should do as much activity as safely possible. Most patients who have had surgery are walking and doing small amounts of activity just hours later because it is good for the body.

Physical Activity for Cancer Prevention

Physical activity is a powerful tool in cancer prevention because nearly everyone can do it. Studies have shown that getting enough exercise can prevent certain cancers. Breast and colon cancer were the first cancers linked to levels of physical activity. Shortly after, studies supported a link between exercise and prevention of endometrial, lung, kidney, and prostate cancers.

A 2016 study published by more than 30 researchers in *JAMA Internal Medicine* explored moderate or vigorous activity completed at the individual's discretion to maintain or improve health. The study looked at 1.4 million adult participants and more than 26 cancer types across the United States and Europe. Thirteen of these cancers showed a decreased risk when individuals were physically active. Data showed a 20% decrease in risk for esophageal **adenocarcinoma** and liver, lung, kidney, gastric, and endometrial cancers, along with **myeloid** leukemia. The study also found a moderate (10%–20%) decrease in multiple myeloma and colorectal, head and neck, bladder, and breast cancers. Overall cancer risk decreased by 7%. Other studies have also shown a decrease in myeloid (blood and bone marrow) cancers with physical activity.

But how does physical activity prevent cancer? Many possible theories exist, as physical activity affects the body in numerous ways. It is thought that **insulin** can trigger cells to multiply out of control. Exercise lowers insulin and insulin-like growth factors, helping to decrease this cell multiplication that can lead to cancer. Activity can reduce fat tissue, central fat, and body mass index, which can also help to lower and regulate hormone levels, as well as increase your energy level. Exercising reduces inflammation and improves immune function. Physical activity could also decrease the amount of time that waste chemicals, which could be cancer-causing, stay in the gastrointestinal system.

Studies have yet to show that exercise early in life prevents more cancer than starting exercise at an older age, proving it is never too late to start. Other studies have shown that not getting enough activity coupled with obesity can increase the risk of breast, kidney, colon, and other digestive cancers. Clearly, physical activity and cancer are linked, and increased activity at all ages benefits overall health and aids in cancer prevention. Staying physically active can also improve symptoms and outcomes for people with cancer. The positive effects of increased activity can grow if combined with other healthy behaviors, such as quitting smoking and eating a healthy diet. Physical activity can play a pivotal role in reducing cancer risk and is something people can control and change. Rarely do we find an intervention that is so powerful and so available to everyone.

Recommendations for Staying Active

Only about half of the adults in the United States and one-third around the world get the recommended 30 minutes of activity most days during the week. Most adults spend most of their waking day sitting in front of the TV or computer. Sitting for more than four hours per day can increase the risk of cancer.

The U.S. Department of Health and Human Services gives clear physical activity guidelines for all ages (see Figure 4-1). The guidelines focus on moderate and vigorous aerobic activity recommendations. *Moderate activity* means working hard enough that talking is possible but singing is not. This includes

Figure 4-1. Examples of Recommended Physical Activity

Moderate Aerobic	Vigorous Aerobic	Muscle Strengthening	Bone Strengthening
• Hiking	• Running	• Push-ups	• Hopscotch
• Brisk walking	• Jogging	• Tug of war	• Skipping
• Most yardwork	• Jumping rope	• Resistance band exercises	• Jumping rope
• Water aerobics	• Most competi-	• Sit-ups	• Running
• Ballroom danc-	tive sports	• Weight lifting	• Basketball
ing	• Swimming laps	• Swinging on	• Tennis
• Skateboarding	• Aerobic danc-	playground	• Volleyball
• Doubles tennis	ing	equipment/bars	
	• Playing tag	• Gymnastics/ cheerleading	

Note. Based on information from Chin, 2014.

things like brisk walking, gardening, and water aerobics. *Vigorous activity* involves working hard enough so that speaking more than a few words is difficult without stopping to take a breath—activities such as swimming laps, jogging, or running. Everyone should engage in regular physical activity that is appropriate based on age and other medical conditions. If you are unsure of what you can do or have a chronic condition, check with your healthcare provider prior to starting any activity (see Figure 4-2).

It is recommended that healthy adults 18–65 years of age complete 150 minutes (2 hours and 30 minutes) of moderate aerobic activity each week or 75 minutes (1 hour and 15 minutes) of vigorous activity each week. Physical activity should be done for at least 10 minutes at a time and be spread out through the week. In addition, healthy adults should complete strength training two days each week. The strength training should include all large muscle groups and 8–12 repetitions of each exercise for those muscle groups. Adults older than age 65 should follow the same guidelines if they are generally healthy. Increased activity for older adults can improve quality of life and decrease risk of developing medical conditions.

Figure 4-2. Recommendations for Physical Activity		
Youths Aged 6–17 Years	**Healthy Adults Aged 18–65 Years**	**Generally Fit Adults Older Than Age 65 Years**
• 1 hour per day of mostly moderate or vigorous aerobic activity • Muscle strengthening and bone strengthening activity at least 3 days per week	• 150 minutes per week of moderate aerobic activity or 75 minutes per week of vigorous activity • 2 days per week of strength training, 8–12 repetitions per muscle group	• Same recommendations as healthy adults • Check with healthcare provider if unsure of safety or if a chronic medical condition exists.

Note. Based on information from Chin, 2014; Office of Disease Prevention and Health Promotion, 2008.

People aged 6–17 also have specific physical activity guidelines. They should have one hour of mostly moderate to vigorous aerobic activity each day. Younger people should also focus their time at least three days of the week on muscle strengthening and bone strengthening activities. The amount of time watching TV or using a computer or smartphone is a large concern for all people but especially for children and teenagers. Recommendations include limiting TV, computer, or smartphone use to less than two hours per day and avoiding prolonged sitting. In fact, sitting for more than four hours per day can actually increase the risk of cancer.

Experts agree that moderate to vigorous activity provides the greatest benefit over light activities. Short, high-intensity regimens tend to provide the best, most sustainable prevention. Increased activity duration, such as 30–60 minutes per day, improves the cancer-preventive effects. Moderate activity is safe for most people, and the benefits outweigh any risks.

If you are not currently physically active, start slowly and gradually increase activity. Talk to your provider before starting exercise if you have long-term health issues. Any activity is better than none, and each person should exercise as vigorously and as safely as possible.

Fitting Physical Activity Into Your Life

Although the evidence clearly supports regular physical activity and its health benefits, people face barriers to being active. Everyone has things that get in the way of doing regular physical activity. The following are common barriers to getting regular exercise:

- Not enough time
- Feeling too tired to exercise (fatigue)
- Family obligations
- Other priorities
- The cost of gym memberships or classes
- No gym close to home or work
- No safe places to walk

One great way to be more active is to set small, attainable goals and gradually increase activity. Self-monitoring tools such as wearable tracking devices, tracking journals, smartphone applications, or pedometers can aid in reaching those goals. Pedometers are especially effective for those who want to achieve 10,000 steps a day, with 3,000 of those being done at a brisk pace. Being active with family and friends also helps; a support system makes exercise easier and more sustainable. Community resources such as walks for different charities or causes, weight loss challenges, local parks, and physical activity groups are other ways to stay active (see Figure 4-3).

Figure 4-3. Tips for Overcoming Barriers to Physical Activity

- Set small, attainable goals to start.
- Use self-monitoring tools: journals, pedometers, or other wearable devices.
- Involve family and friends.
- Use community resources.
- Get up and move at least every hour while working.
- Take the stairs instead of the elevator.
- Park farther away from an entrance.
- Walk during lunch breaks.

Note. Based on information from AuYoung et al., 2016; Chin, 2014; Lemanne et al., 2013; National Institutes of Health, 2016.

Working all day makes it very difficult for many people to find time for physical activity. Several tips and tricks can help people fit in activity throughout the day. Use a timer to remind yourself to get up at least once an hour. When the timer goes off, climb one or two flights of stairs, stretch, or take a short walk. Stand up and move around during phone calls to avoid sitting all day. In addition, treadmill desks and standing desks may assist in avoiding sitting all day. If meetings run long, take a break for a quick walk, or walk during a lunch break. Many companies even offer exercise classes, workout rooms, or gym discounts for employees.

Small and simple things often add physical activity to the day. Parking farther away from a building entrance or taking the stairs instead of the elevator can contribute to that 10,000-step goal. Everyday housework, such as raking leaves and other yardwork, also counts as physical activity. Remember, any activity is better than no activity. Some activity can double as time to unwind; a walk, rowing, or hiking can be relaxing while maintaining fitness levels. Use activity as a reward rather than an obligation. Finally, keeping screen time to a minimum will increase overall health and decrease mortality. About 90% of U.S. older adults watch 4.7 hours of television per day. Fitting in some activity during commercials is an easy way to lessen the negative effects of sitting for such a long time when watching television.

FACT OR FICTION: Just taking the stairs won't provide much benefit.

Fiction. Taking the stairs instead of elevators or escalators can benefit your health. It burns three times as many calories as briskly walking and seven times as many calories as riding the elevator. It can also increase the chances of weight loss. Walking only two flights of stairs a day can lead to a 2- to 6-pound weight loss each year. Climbing the stairs increases your heart rate and blood flow, which helps your heart, and it also helps to tone muscles.

Summary

People want the most for their money, and physical activity certainly provides a large "bang for your buck" when it comes to health. Everyone can exercise, even in small increments. Unfortunately, according to a 2016 study in *JAMA Internal Medicine*, only 50% of U.S. adults meet aerobic exercise guidelines, and only 24% meet the strength-training guidelines. Although exercise is powerful for improving health and preventing cancer, only 20% of U.S. adults meet both the aerobic and strength-training activity recommendations. It is important to take control and exercise regularly not only to prevent certain cancers but also for the overlap of improvement in other diseases. Maintaining physical activity can decrease the risk of dying from many conditions. Although research shows that increasing activity can prevent some cancers, more studies are necessary to show its true effect on all cancer types. That said, people of all ages should incorporate physical activity to improve quality of life and overall health.

Recommended Reading

American Cancer Society. (2016). ACS guidelines on nutrition and physical activity for cancer prevention. Retrieved from https://www.cancer.org/healthy/eat-healthy-get-active/acs-guidelines-nutrition-physical-activity-cancer-prevention.html

Centers for Disease Control and Prevention. (2015). Physical activity and health: The benefits of physical activity. Retrieved from https://www.cdc.gov/physicalactivity/basics/pa-health/index.htm

National Cancer Institute. (2017). Physical activity and cancer. Retrieved from https://www.cancer.gov/about-cancer/causes-prevention/risk/obesity/physical-activity-fact-sheet

National Institutes of Health. (2016). Physical activity and your heart. Retrieved from https://www.nhlbi.nih.gov/book/export/html/4853

Office of Disease Prevention and Health Promotion. (2017). Physical activity guidelines for Americans. Retrieved from https://health.gov/paguidelines/guidelines

Glossary

adenocarcinoma [ad-e-noh-kahr-suh-noh-muh]—A malignant tumor arising from secretory epithelium; a malignant tumor of a gland-like structure.

insulin—Hormone produced by the pancreas that helps the body metabolize carbohydrates, fats, and proteins and regulates blood sugar.

myeloid—Relating to bone marrow.

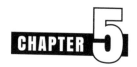

CHAPTER 5

Food and Nutrition

Jane Taylor Williams, MSN, RN, FNP-BC

> *Let food be thy medicine and medicine be thy food.*
> —Hippocrates

Proper diet, regular physical activity, and weight management may prevent many cancers (see Figure 5-1). The U.S. Burden of Disease Collaborators ranked dietary risks as the highest among 17 leading factors that contribute to death and disability in the United States. Diets low in fruits, vegetables, whole grains, nuts and seeds, milk, fiber, calcium, and seafood contribute to this risk. Diets high in red meat, processed meats, sugar-sweetened beverages, trans fats, and sodium also add to health risks. In addition to the type of diet we consume, weight management is also important. The American Institute for Cancer Research (AICR) estimates that approximately 3.2% of new cancer cases are linked to obesity, and overweight and obesity con-

---

Figure 5-1. Overweight and Obesity Increase the Risk for These Cancers

- Advanced prostate cancer
- Colorectal cancer
- Endometrial cancer
- Esophageal cancer
- Gallbladder cancer
- Kidney cancer
- Liver cancer
- Ovarian cancer
- Pancreatic cancer
- Postmenopausal breast cancer
- Stomach cancer

---

tributes to 14%–20% of all cancer-related deaths. Nearly 38% of adults and 17% of children and adolescents are obese in the United States, and the prevalence has risen astonishingly over the past few decades. A 2016 report from the Centers for Disease Control and Prevention showed that more Americans had health insurance and fewer smoked cigarettes than in previous years; however, they found the rate of obesity rose from 2014 and has consistently risen since at least 1997.

Food is meant to nourish; it is necessary for life, health, and growth. Food is also meant to be enjoyed and is a way of caring for ourselves and others. Food is a part of life's celebrations, including birthdays, graduations, weddings, anniversaries, holidays, and more. Some people find artistic expression in preparing and serving food, and it also connects us to the environment. However, sometimes to care for or comfort ourselves, the foods we choose only provide a brief psychological benefit and no physical benefit. Instead, they may be harmful. Unfortunately, more than 50% of calories in the typical Western diet come from foods with refined sugars, bleached flour, excess salt, and unhealthy vegetable oils. These foods contain few nutrients, promote inflammation, and increase the risk of obesity and insulin resistance. This, in turn, increases the risk for not only cancer but also for heart disease, diabetes, and Alzheimer disease.

The Benefits of Healthy Foods

Plant foods contain more than a thousand different **phytonutrients**—natural chemicals found in plants, similar to vitamins and minerals. Research shows they protect against all types of diseases, including cancer. The foods we eat may alter genetic expression, and some phytonutrients work together with chemotherapy and radiation. These bioactive compounds may inhibit formation of carcinogens. Antioxidants protect the body from damage caused by harmful molecules called *free radicals*. They include some vitamins, some minerals, and flavonoids, which are found in plants. The best sources of antioxidants are vegetables and fruits. Antioxidants may prevent tumor initiation, and other nutrients may repair damaged genes or regulate the immune system. Scientists continue to study these compounds to better understand which are most beneficial. Until more is known, the medical community recommends eating a wide variety of plants for cancer prevention—many types and colors of vegetables and fruits.

What to Eat

AICR recommends the following guidelines for nutrition:
- Avoid sugary drinks (soft drinks, sweetened tea).
- Limit consumption of energy-dense (high-calorie) foods.
- Eat a variety of vegetables, fruits, whole grains, and **legumes**.
- Limit consumption of red meats (beef, pork, lamb) and avoid processed meats (hot dogs, pepperoni and other similar meats, lunch meats).
- If consumed at all, limit alcoholic drinks to two per day for men and one per day for women. (One drink equals 12 fluid ounces of beer, 5 fluid ounces of wine, or 1.5 fluid ounces of hard liquor.)
- Limit consumption of salty foods and foods processed with salt.
- Don't use supplements to protect against cancer.

A Whole-Food, Plant-Based Diet

The American Cancer Society (ACS) and AICR recommend a whole-food, plant-based diet that does not exclude animal products. A plant-based diet means at least two-thirds of the plate should be filled with plant foods. Plant-based foods include vegetables, fruits, whole grains, legumes, nuts, and seeds. Eating a whole-food diet means most of the foods we choose should be as nature made them—unaltered, unprocessed, a single ingredient—such as an apple, broccoli, black beans, or an egg. Whole foods optimize nutritional content, limit empty calories, and avoid artificial ingredients and preservatives. Eating these types of foods also provides synergy of the nutrients, meaning together they provide more nutrition than from individual nutrients alone.

Processed foods (boxed, bagged, and jarred) have few nutrients and include added sugar, salt, unhealthy oils, artificial ingredients, and preservatives.

Vegetables and Fruits

ACS recommends at least 5 servings of vegetables and fruits per day but further recommends that women eat 5–9 servings and men eat 7–11 servings, so try to include vegetables or fruits at every meal. See Table 5-1 for serving sizes. Adding fruit, such as berries, oranges, and bananas, to breakfast offers a nutritious way to start the day. Scrambled eggs or an omelet with a variety of vegetables, such as spinach, mushrooms, tomatoes, bell peppers, and scallions, is another satisfying breakfast. Drinking fruit juice may be more palatable, but some juices, such as apple juice, may be little more than sugar water. Using a blender rather than a juicer to make a blended drink provides the nutrients and fiber of the whole fruit, which is beneficial for cancer prevention. When it comes to side dishes, salads and roasted vegetables provide more nutrients than french fries or chips. Snacks of fruit plus a protein, such as berries and plain Greek yogurt or an apple and almond butter, satisfy cravings just as well as candy bars or chips without added calories.

Table 5-1. What Is a Serving Size?	
Food	**Serving Size**
Raw vegetables or fruits	1 cup coarsely chopped, or 1 piece of whole fruit (apple, orange) the size of a baseball or a small fist
Cooked or canned vegetables or fruits	½ cup
Dried fruit, no added sugar, no preservatives	2–4 tablespoons
Fruit or vegetable juice, 100% juice, no added sugar	4 ounces (½ cup) or small juice glass; limit to one serving per day

Both raw and cooked vegetables have specific benefits. Some nutrients are more abundant when cooked, such as lycopene in tomatoes. Other nutrients, such as beta-carotene in carrots and other water-soluble vitamins, may be diminished when boiled. However, the leftover cooking liquid can be used to cook rice or pasta. Sautéing in oil may increase the availability of some beneficial fat-soluble phytochemicals. In general, cooking breaks down plant cell walls and makes nutrients and other phytochemicals more readily available. Fresh or frozen vegetables and fruits are preferred over canned because canned varieties may have added salt or sugar. However, canned fruits or vegetables are still preferable to none, especially if cost is a factor. Consider buying organic rather than conventional, if available and if the cost is not a burden; some pesticides and herbicides have been found to increase the risk of cancer, and organic produce is grown without them. You should wash all fruits and vegetables, especially non-organic produce, to rid them of the pesticides and bacteria. Remember, the benefit of eating vegetables and fruits outweighs the risk of eating non-organic. The Environmental Working Group publishes lists of the "Clean Fifteen" and "Dirty Dozen" fruits and vegetables with the most and least pesticide residue, as well as other guidelines on pesticides, on its website (www.ewg.org), updated annually.

Legumes

Eating legumes such as beans, peas, soybeans, and lentils frequently may help you maintain a healthy weight. They are an excellent source of fiber, lean protein, minerals, antioxidants, and other phytonutrients. Legumes can substitute for meat, such as a black bean burger instead of ground beef, a vegetable chili with beans instead of ground meat, lentil stew with eggplant or other vegetables, or a tofu and vegetable stir-fry instead of pork or chicken. Each type of bean varies in the amount and type of antioxidants and other nutrients, so eating a variety offers the most benefit.

Soybeans and soy products contain genistein, a phytoestrogen (plant-based estrogen), which binds estrogen receptors to slow cancer growth. Soy is a complete protein, meaning it has all the essential amino acids (building blocks of proteins) that humans need. Like other beans, soybeans are a good source of fiber and minerals such as magnesium, copper, manganese, and iron. Soy-based products like soy milk and tofu contain added calcium. Studies have shown that certain soy products such as edamame (immature soybeans), tofu, miso, tempeh, and soy milk may even be beneficial to women who have estrogen receptor–positive breast cancer. Other soy products made with soy isolates or soy isoflavones—soy protein powders, soy protein energy bars, or soy burgers and other soy-based meat substitutes—are often high-dose extracts, which can be harmful. Because they are pro-estrogenic, they may increase the risk of endometrial, breast, ovarian, and bladder cancers. They may also increase the risk of kidney stones, diabetes, underactive thyroid, and asthma.

Whole Grains

Choosing whole grains over simple grains is beneficial (see Figure 5-2). A 2016 **meta-analysis** found that people who eat whole grains regularly, approximately three servings per day, have a lower risk for all causes of death, including cancer. Whole grains are high in fiber, have more protein than simple grains, and contain greater levels of vitamins and other nutrients. Adding whole grains to your diet is easy because they come in a wide variety, such as oatmeal or steel-cut oats, brown or wild rice (or a blend), whole-grain cereals and breads, whole-wheat pasta, hulled barley, quinoa, and buckwheat. Try cooking unfamiliar whole grains in low-sodium chicken broth or vegetable broth for more flavor until you are more used to eating them. Adding vegetables such as sliced asparagus, onions, or shredded brussels sprouts to quinoa makes it more flavorful. Searching the Internet for recipes can help you add variety to meals. Everyone should reduce the amount of simple or refined grains they eat, such as white bread, white rice, white pasta, crackers, and sugars. Processing grains strips them of fiber and vitamins. Food manufacturers often enrich these foods by adding artificial vitamins. By reading food

Figure 5-2. Whole Versus Simple Grains		
Whole Grains (eat more)	**Simple Grains (eat less)**	**Gluten-Free Grains (eat if sensitive to wheat)**
• Amaranth • Brown or wild rice • Buckwheat or kasha (toasted buckwheat) • Farro • Hulled barley • Kamut • Millet • Oatmeal or steel-cut oats • Quinoa • Sorghum • Spelt • Whole-grain cereals and breads • Whole-wheat pasta	• White crackers • White flour • White pasta • White rice • White sugars	• Amaranth • Brown or wild rice • Buckwheat or kasha (toasted buckwheat) • Millet • Oatmeal or steel-cut oats • Quinoa • Sorghum

labels, you can determine if the product is mostly whole wheat or whole grain versus white or enriched flour. Reading food labels also helps you to determine the amount of added sugars. The typical Western diet is full of simple grains. These foods may cause frequent spikes and dips in blood sugar throughout the day, which is an inflammatory process and can increase the risk of cancer and other diseases, a topic discussed in more detail in Chapter 8. Eating simple grains occasionally will only temporarily raise the blood sugar and will not create an inflammatory process.

Oils and Fats

Our bodies need both omega-3 and omega-6 fats. However, the ratio of the two types of fats is important for managing inflammation. Omega-3 fats help reduce inflammation in the body, but omega-6 fats increase inflammation. Therefore, people should eat more foods high in omega-3s and fewer foods high in omega-6s (see Figure 5-3).

Olive and canola oils are healthy for cooking. However, these oils should not be used at high temperatures. For higher-heat

---

Figure 5-3. Omega-3 and Omega-6 Foods

Omega-3 Rich Foods (eat more)
- Avocados, olives
- Meat, dairy, and eggs from grass-fed or pasture-raised animals
- Olive oil, canola oil, avocado oil, walnut oil
- Walnuts, pecans, cashews, ground flaxseed, chia seeds, pumpkin seeds
- Wild-caught, cold-water fish: black cod, halibut, herring, mackerel, salmon, sardines, tuna

Omega-6 Rich Foods (eat less)
- Deep-fried fish, meat, or vegetables
- Meat and full-fat dairy from grain-fed animals
- Peanuts, sunflower seeds
- Soybean oil, corn oil, peanut oil, hydrogenated oil, or trans fats (often found in processed foods)
- Tilapia

---

cooking such as stir-frying, a high-oleic grape-seed oil is preferable. Because of its anti-inflammatory properties, coconut oil is great for making muffins or pancakes (using whole-grain flour and low-glycemic sweeteners such as agave nectar or stevia). The oils in avocados and most nuts are also healthy dietary options.

Nuts and Seeds

Most nuts and seeds contain healthy fats as well as fiber, antioxidants, and other nutrients. However, they are high in calories and fat and therefore should be eaten in small amounts, approximately one-fourth cup each day, to avoid possible weight gain. Walnuts and pecans contain high levels of omega-3 fats, whereas peanuts are higher in omega-6 fats. Pistachios are a good source of antioxidants. Choosing raw or dry-roasted varieties avoids added fat and calories.

Fermented Foods

Fermented foods naturally add live and active cultures, or probiotics, to the diet while also adding flavor and variety. Probiotics are bacteria and yeasts that keep a natural balance of organisms (microflora) in the intestines. The normal human digestive tract contains about 400 types of probiotic bacteria that reduce the growth of harmful bacteria and promote a healthy digestive system. A decrease in beneficial bacteria may lead to other health problems. Probiotics are being studied for potential cancer risk reduction of colon and other cancers, but the medical community still has much to learn. Dairy products such as plain Greek yogurt or kefir (liquid yogurt) offer probiotic benefits, as do sauerkraut (found in the refrigerated section), kimchi (fermented vegetables in spices), miso (fermented soy used in soups), and kombucha (fermented tea).

Animal Products

Remember that a serving of meat should take up no more than one-third of a standard dinner plate. When choosing meat products, limit the amount of red meat—beef, pork, lamb, goat, buffalo, venison, and elk. Recent studies have found that red meat in large amounts can increase the risk of cancer because of a sugar molecule called Neu5Gc found in most mammals, except humans. Therefore, humans develop an inflammatory response to eating red meat. ACS recommends 18 ounces or less of red meat each week. Dairy products do not contain this sugar molecule. ACS also recommends limiting processed meats such as hot dogs, pepperoni, ham, bacon, sausage, and sliced sandwich meats. These foods contain preservative chemicals that increase cancer risk. Many grocery stores now offer preservative-free, or nitrate-/nitrite-free, sandwich meat options.

On the other hand, poultry, fish, and shellfish have not been linked with increased cancer risk. When buying meat, choosing lean cuts and removing the skin from chicken or other fowl are the best options. When grilling meats, cook on lower temperatures and place meats to the side so they are not directly over the flame because grilling meats may produce carcinogens when the fats drip on the hot coals. Using marinades made with vinegar or lemon juice may reduce the levels of carcinogens. After cooking, remove and discard any charred or blackened portions prior to eating.

You may want to reduce dairy products in your diet, especially high-fat varieties. Soft cheeses and 2% milk are healthier alternatives to hard cheeses and whole milk. Plain Greek yogurt, which has more protein and active cultures, is another healthy alternative. Adding fruit and a low-glycemic sweetener, like agave nectar, enhances the yogurt without adding many calories. You should choose dairy products that have no added growth hormones, such as rBGH, which has been implicated in hormone-derived cancers, such as breast, ovarian, and prostate cancers. Organic dairy products usually do not use synthetic growth hormones.

Eggs can also be a healthy addition to a diet. They contain approximately 6 grams of protein and approximately 13 essential vitamins and minerals—vitamins A, D, B_6, B_{12}, riboflavin, and folate, as well as the minerals iron, phosphorus, zinc, and calcium.

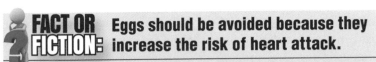

FACT OR FICTION? Eggs should be avoided because they increase the risk of heart attack.

Fiction. Contrary to previous beliefs, eggs do not contribute to high cholesterol levels or heart disease.

Salt

The U.S. Food and Drug Administration advises limiting salt consumption to 2,400 mg, or about 1 teaspoon, per day. Most processed foods are high in salt, so limit the amount you eat. Avoid snacks like chips, fries, and pretzels, and be aware of high sodium content in canned soups, frozen meals, breads, and even some desserts. Carefully reading food labels reveals the sodium content. When buying products such as canned tomatoes, soups, and broths, choose varieties with little or no added salt. Rinsing canned vegetables prior to heating removes much of the added salt. Add less salt while cooking and preparing meals, and season with herbs and spices instead.

Sweeteners

Some artificial sweeteners, such as saccharin (Sweet'N Low®), sucralose (Splenda®), and aspartame and acesulfame potassium (found in Equal®), may increase cancer risk, so it is important to be judicious when using them. They may also contribute to increased appetite, cravings for additional sweet foods, and weight gain. Many sugar-free and reduced-calorie products contain these artificial sweeteners.

Diets should limit simple sugars including table sugar, brown sugar, powdered sugar, raw sugar, and turbinado sugar, which contribute to the inflammation caused by frequent spikes and dips in blood sugars. Read food labels to look for other sources of sugar such as cane juice, corn syrup, high-fructose corn syrup, molasses, glucose, polydextrose, or fructose. Honey and maple syrup may be slightly better options as they are minimally processed and contain small amounts of vitamins and minerals. However, they can cause spikes in blood sugar, too, so use them in small amounts for flavoring only. Gradually reducing sugar in foods and beverages will help you get used to the different taste.

Instead of the sweeteners previously mentioned, low-glycemic sweeteners are better options, such as coconut palm sugar, agave nectar, and stevia, a natural, no-calorie sweetener.

Other Foods

Don't forget to add a little spice to life. Using herbs and spices increases flavor and can help you limit excess salt. Spices such as turmeric (curcumin) or ginger may provide an anti-inflammatory benefit, while herbs such as oregano, thyme, basil, rosemary, and parsley can provide antioxidants. Experimenting with a variety of herbs and spices can inject a little excitement into a diet.

Green or black teas also provide antioxidants. Green tea extract has been implicated in liver toxicity because of the high concentration of one antioxidant. Based on recommendations, you should limit consumption to two cups per day. Coffee contains antioxidants as well, but a limit of two cups per day avoids caffeine-related sleep disturbances. Dark chocolate with at least 70% cacao contains little sugar, has antioxidants, and increases our natural oxytocin levels that make us feel good. This may satisfy a sweet tooth without adding too much sugar.

Dietary Supplements

ACS and AICR recommend avoiding supplements for cancer prevention. No single vitamin or mineral has consistently shown any benefits for the prevention of cancer unless a person has a dietary deficiency, which is uncommon in the United States. Some vitamins may increase the risk for cancer development. Because supplements are unregulated, manufacturers can put virtually anything in the products, including only fillers. Dr. Tim Byers from the University of Colorado presented his meta-analysis research in which he found a number of supplements actually increased the risk of developing certain types of cancers. His sentiment is a good mantra: "There is no substitute for good, nutritional food."

Weight Management

Managing weight is important to overall health, and it should be accomplished safely. If you are overweight or obese, even a loss of 5% of total weight can significantly improve your overall health and reduce your risk of cancer and other diseases. Weight loss decreases cancer risk by lowering estrogen, insulin, glucose, and C-reactive protein, which is a measure of inflammation. It may also lower your risk of other diseases such as high blood pressure, diabetes, and heart disease. When attempting to lose weight, eating right matters. You can achieve the most sustainable weight loss gradually by eating healthier foods and incorporating them into your regular eating habits.

Food Journal

Keeping a food journal aids in recognizing food portions, unhealthy choices, and perhaps even emotional triggers—reasons why you eat. A food journal helps us to face what we are feeling when we want to make that 4 pm trip to the vending machine every day or when we grab a bag of cookies after an emotional encounter. Along with a journal, using the acronym "HALT" helps us understand if we are hungry, angry, lonely, or tired. We can then work to find alternate solutions in dealing with our real sources of perceived hunger.

Mindfulness

Mindful eating is being aware of *how* we eat. Eating too fast and mindlessly often eliminates enjoyment and satisfaction, which leads to seeking additional servings to get the pleasure of eating. Taking time to appreciate the qualities of food—colors, texture, and aroma—and thinking about what the food feels and tastes like automatically slows down eating, so we can savor and enjoy our meal. Ultimately, the brain more quickly recognizes the stomach's message of fullness, thus reducing unnecessary eating.

Being mindful also is a way of planning and choosing what we eat and how we prepare our food. Making grocery lists before shopping makes following the nutrition guidelines previously mentioned easier. Once at the store, shop only for items on the list, rather than perusing each aisle with the chance of being lured to unhealthy choices.

Eating at Home

Cooking at home is the best option to know what is in your food and how it is prepared. If your daily schedule limits your ability to cook full meals, look for quick and simple recipes. You can prepare extra portions, especially on days off when you have more time, so you have leftover meals to freeze for later. If you buy frozen entrees, remember to read food labels and make healthy choices. Some grocery stores sell freshly prepared meals, but choose wisely here also. Many cities have businesses that sell healthy options for convenient takeout foods.

It also helps when the entire family agrees to eat at home more often rather than at restaurants. Family members can participate in planning, shopping, and cooking. Even if a family member can only chop, open containers, or stir, he or she feels involved and can enjoy participating. Young family members can help with setting the table and retrieving items from the refrigerator or pantry. Encouraging children to grow vegetables or herbs, even in small containers, involves them in food preparation and establishes pride in growing something nutritious they can eat.

Summary

Evidence shows that good nutrition and maintaining a normal weight can reduce the risk of many cancers and other diseases. What we eat matters; therefore, we should follow a whole-food, plant-based diet that includes a wide variety of vegetables, fruits, legumes, whole grains, healthy oils, and healthy animal products. Foods to limit include simple grains, sugars, unhealthy oils, red meats, processed meats, and other processed foods. Also limit alcohol, salty foods, artificial sweeteners, and other artificial ingredients. Involving the entire family makes this easier and more enjoyable. Remember to be mindful when planning meals, shopping, and eating. A balanced diet can be both nutritious and satisfying.

Recommended Reading

American Institute for Cancer Research. (n.d.). Recommendations for cancer prevention. Retrieved from http://www.aicr.org/reduce-your-cancer-risk/recommendations-for-cancer-prevention

Environmental Working Group. (2017). Executive summary: EWG's 2017 shopper's guide to pesticides in produce. Retrieved from https://www.ewg.org/foodnews/summary.php

Katz, R., & Edelson, M. (2017). *The cancer-fighting kitchen: Nourishing, big-flavor recipes for cancer treatment and recovery* (2nd ed.). Berkeley, CA: Ten Speed Press.

Kushi, L.H., Doyle, C., McCullough, M., Rock, C.L., Demark-Wahnefried, W., Bandera, E.V., ... Gansler, T. (2012). American Cancer Society guidelines on nutrition and physical activity for cancer prevention: Reducing the risk of cancer with healthy food choices and physical activity. *CA: A Cancer Journal for Clinicians, 62*, 30–67. doi:10.3322/caac.20140

Sundem, G. (2015, April 20). Dietary supplements shown to increase cancer risk. *Colorado Cancer Blogs*. Retrieved from http://www.coloradocancerblogs.org/dietary-supplements-shown-to-increase-cancer-risk

Zong, G., Gao, A., Hu, F.B., & Sun, Q. (2016). Whole grain intake and mortality from all causes, cardiovascular disease, and cancer: A meta-analysis

of prospective cohort studies. *Circulation, 133,* 2370–2380. doi:10.1161/
CIRCULATIONAHA.115.021101

Glossary

legume [leg-yoom]—The large plant family *Leguminosae* (or *Fabaceae*), typi-
fied by herbaceous plants, shrubs, trees, and vines having usually compound leaves, clusters of irregular, keeled flowers, and fruit in the form of
a pod splitting along both sides, and including beans, peas, acacia, alfalfa,
clover, indigo, lentil, mesquite, mimosa, and peanut.

meta-analysis—A process that analyzes data from different studies done
about the same subject. The results of a meta-analysis are usually stronger
than the results of any study by itself.

phytonutrient [fahy-tuh-noo-tree-uhnt]—Any of the various bioactive chemical compounds found in plants, such as antioxidants, considered to be
beneficial to human health.

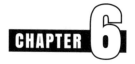

CHAPTER 6

Alcohol and Tobacco

Andrew S. Guinigundo, MSN, RN, CNP, ANP-BC

> *Vice [vīs]—Noun. An immoral or evil habit or practice; a fault, defect, or shortcoming; a bad habit.*

I *propose a toast. Prost! Salud! Sláinte! Santé! Salute! Cheers!* No matter how you say it, drinking alcoholic beverages is part of everyday life for many. The National Institute on Alcohol Abuse and Alcoholism (NIAAA) reported that 71% of Americans aged 18 years and older have had a drink in the past year. Nearly 25% have participated in binge drinking—consuming the amount of alcohol required to raise your blood alcohol level to the level of legal intoxication. Alcoholism, also known as alcohol use disorder, goes beyond how many drinks a person has. It also includes how mentally and physically dependent a person is on alcohol and how it affects that person's life. NIAAA estimated that more than 16 million adults aged 18 years and older had an alcohol use disorder in 2014. Shockingly, 679,000 youths aged 12–17 years had an alcohol use disorder in 2014.

Smoke 'em if you got 'em. Let's take a smoke break. These days, smoking is perhaps not as socially acceptable as it once was. However, the American Lung Association (ALA) noted only a 7% decrease in smoking between 1965 and 2009. Although this decrease may not seem like a big deal, there is a silver lining. Social changes such as prohibiting smoking in public places (bars and restaurants), removal of unmonitored cigarette vending machines, movie ratings taking a film's inclusion of smoking into account, and the increased knowledge of bad health effects of smoking may be influencing this decrease. The 2014 U.S. Department of Health and Human Services Surgeon General's report on smoking concluded that programs designed to curb smoking, even dating back to the original report on smoking in 1964, have made an impact on the number of people smoking. ALA also notes the number of former smokers has jumped considerably—from 24 million in 1965 to nearly 52 million in 2009.

Whether one defines a vice as an immoral and evil act or simply a bad habit, alcohol consumption and tobacco use are part of our society. Using these products as intended, even in small amounts, can lead to health problems, even cancer.

Why We Like Alcohol and Tobacco

Alcohol

Alcohol is classified as a depressant. Even at low levels, it can decrease coordination, attention, and clear thinking. At higher levels, it can cause impaired judgment, slurred speech, nausea and vomiting, and impaired walking or driving. Of course, none of these explain why people would want to take such a drug, as none of those effects seem desirable.

Alcohol produces desirable euphoria, meaning it makes us feel good. People also enjoy an aged liquor, a fine wine, or a craft beer simply because it tastes good. That euphoria keeps the booze pouring and can lead to addiction.

We may be "born" to ingest alcohol, and the reason could be in our DNA. Evolutionary biology studies how species have changed, sometimes over millions of years, to adapt to where they live and other environmental factors. In the book *The Drunken Monkey: Why We Drink and Abuse Alcohol*, evolutionary biologist Robert Dudley from the University of California theorized that our monkey ancestors may have been very good at figuring out the best ripeness of fruit, which is the time the fruit has the most calories. These primates may have done this by smelling the scent of sugar and the small amounts of natural alcohol in that fruit. Fast-forward to today, and we may still have the drive to chase that high-calorie food. However, the extent of our hunting and gathering involves jumping in the car, running to the market, and grabbing a six-pack of beer to share. More proof comes from researchers who studied samples of ADH4, an alcohol-metabolizing enzyme found in primates that had existed for more than 50 million years. They saw a change in the enzyme, occurring about 10 million years ago, that made it break down alcohol more effectively. They believe this change allowed primates to leave the trees and live on the ground. They could eat fruit that had fallen to the ground and contained more alcohol and more calories. This evolutionary change occurred millions of years before any human-directed alcohol production, such as brewing beer, took place. Humans making alcohol only dates back about 9,000 years.

Tobacco

Nicotine, the addictive drug in tobacco, is a stimulant that relaxes the user. According to the American Cancer Society, nicotine causes happy feelings while also reducing unhappy feelings. The American Cancer Society indicates nicotine gives users a small adrenaline rush—not enough to be noticed but enough to cause increased heart rate and blood pressure. Nicotine reaches the brain within seconds of a person taking a puff on a cigarette. This stimulates a chemical called dopamine to flood the brain, creating that feeling of happiness. This recurring feeling can quickly lead to addiction.

The tobacco plant is native to North and South America, and the leaves become the various forms of tobacco that people use. The plant began to grow around 6000 BC, and Native Americans first used tobacco for religious and medicinal purposes around 1 BC. In 1492, when Christopher Columbus landed in the Americas, he received dried tobacco leaves as a gift. Not long after, tobacco was brought to Europe and grown there. Into the 20th century, cigarettes gained popularity as soldiers embraced smoking during World War I. During World War II, American soldiers were given cigarettes in their ration packs, and many soldiers received free cigarettes from tobacco companies. Returning soldiers became loyal, lifetime smokers. According to the Surgeon General's report on smoking, these factors, along with advertising downplaying health risks and a lack of laws prohibiting smoking in public, led to smoking's social acceptance in the mid-20th century.

Often, smoking addiction starts early in life. According to the Surgeon General's report, 87% of people who had ever smoked daily tried their first cigarette by age 18, and 14% of adults who had ever smoked daily first smoked before they started high school.

Alcohol- and Tobacco-Related Health Issues

Alcohol

According to NIAAA, alcohol affects the body in numerous ways. Excessive use can cause changing mood, behavior, movement, and thinking. Alcohol can cause cardiovascular problems, such as **cardiomyopathy** (heart muscle disease), irregular heartbeat, strokes, and high blood pressure. The American Heart Association mentions these risks and adds that too much drinking can increase bad fat, such as triglycerides, in the body. Extra calories associated with drinking can lead to obesity and diabetes, too. These factors all increase the risk for heart issues. NIAAA warns that alcohol can cause pancreatitis—inflammation of the pancreas—leading to improper digestion and stomach pain. Chapter 8 discusses inflammation as a cancer risk factor in detail. Excessive and chronic alcohol consumption weakens the immune system and can make the drinker more susceptible to infection for up to 24 hours after drinking.

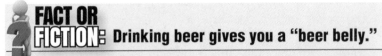

FACT OR FICTION: Drinking beer gives you a "beer belly."

Fact. In general, taking in more calories than you expend causes fat to be deposited throughout your body. As we age, more fat tends to accumulate in our midsections. The average beer has 150 calories, quickly adding up to some serious caloric intake and easily creating a potbelly if you're not physically active.

Finally, the American Liver Foundation reports liver issues associated with alcohol in three major categories: fatty liver disease, alcoholic hepatitis, and alcoholic cirrhosis. Fatty liver disease occurs when too much fat builds up within the liver. It is the earliest sign of alcohol-related liver disease. It can lead to fatigue, weakness, and weight loss. Alcoholic hepatitis is an inflammation of the liver that leads to liver damage. More than one-third of heavy drinkers may develop this form of hepatitis. Mild cases can be reversed. Severe cases can lead to liver failure and death. According to the American Liver Foundation, symptoms may include loss of appetite, nausea and vomiting, abdominal pain, fever, and jaundice (yellowing of skin and eyes). The final category of alcoholic liver damage is the most severe—alcoholic cirrhosis. With cirrhosis, scar tissue replaces healthy liver tissue because of long-term damage, with symptoms similar to hepatitis. Although stopping drinking can prevent additional damage, the condition is irreversible.

Tobacco

Much has been written about the health hazards of tobacco. A long-term research study followed 1,711 men for 35 years, and results showed a death rate 84% higher for smokers than nonsmokers. Encouragingly, the study found that former smokers had a death rate equal to that of nonsmokers. Regarding heart disease specifically, the news is grim. Another study noted a 2.35 times higher risk of heart disease in men who smoked 15 or more cigarettes per day versus male nonsmokers. In women, the numbers were even more dramatic. Women who smoked 15 or more cigarettes per day had a 4.85 times greater risk of heart disease than nonsmoking women. Combining information from eight other studies, this study analyzed the information of nearly 300,000 participants. Although a direct connection between smoking and cardiovascular disease has been confirmed, the exact part that cigarette smoke plays in heart issues remains to be completely understood.

The most popular form of tobacco today is cigarette smoking, which can lead to lung diseases other than cancer, including chronic obstructive pulmonary disease (COPD). ALA defines COPD as a lung disease that makes it hard to breathe over time. Cigarette smoking causes about 90% of COPD cases. ALA states, "The toxins in cigarette smoke weaken your lungs' defense against infections, narrow air passages, cause swelling in air tubes and destroy air sacs—all contributing factors for COPD." See Figure 6-1 for ALA's key points on COPD. The most recent Surgeon General's report confirmed these facts by examining 50 years of data regarding smoking and COPD since the first Surgeon General's report in 1964. The report states that enough information exists to conclude that smoking is the main cause of COPD in the United States. More recently, the number of women dying from COPD has surpassed that of men. The U.S. Department of Health and Human Services stated, "Smoking avoidance will remain the key primary prevention approach for COPD, but for the millions of already affected individuals, translation of advances . . . will provide important challenges for decades to come."

Figure 6-1. Chronic Obstructive Pulmonary Disease: Key Points

• COPD is sometimes referred to as chronic bronchitis or emphysema.
• COPD is chronic. In other words, you live with it every day.
• It can cause serious, long-term disability and early death.
• There is no cure for COPD, but it is often preventable and treatable.

Note. Based on information from American Lung Association, 2016.

Alcohol, Tobacco, and Cancer

Alcohol

A large amount of research points to an increased risk of cancer related to alcohol consumption. Since 2000, the National

Toxicology Program has listed alcohol as a known carcinogen. In addition, the National Cancer Institute (NCI) has reviewed the available information on alcohol and cancer. They concluded that the following cancers were most closely linked to alcohol consumption: head and neck (mostly oral cavity, throat, and **larynx**), esophageal, liver, breast, and colon cancer.

The International Agency for Research on Cancer (IARC) in association with the World Health Organization examined alcohol and cancer research and reported their findings in a 1,440-page report. Regarding head and neck cancer, people who consume about 3.5 drinks per day saw triple the risk for oral and throat cancer and double the risk for cancer of the larynx (voice box) over nondrinkers. The risk was even higher in those who were both drinkers and smokers. Drinking the same amount led to double the chances for esophageal cancer, with 50 research studies all pointing to this connection. Based on firm evidence, alcohol intake can also lead to liver cancer. However, putting a number on the risk is difficult because many will develop cirrhosis and quit or slow drinking before they get liver cancer.

Some newer additions to the IARC report include information on female breast cancer and colon cancer. The report examined 58,000 women across 100 studies. A clear relationship between the degree of alcohol consumption and breast cancer exists, suggesting the more alcohol a woman drinks, the more likely she is to get breast cancer. A woman who drinks three drinks per day is 1.5 times more likely to develop breast cancer than a nondrinker. Even consuming as little as 1.3 drinks per day was associated with a 13% increase in breast cancer. In fact, a more recent United Kingdom study noted that for each 10-gram increase in alcohol consumption beyond three drinks, researchers saw an 11% increase in cancer risk. This is less than one drink as defined in the United States. This association does not appear to be related to other risk factors of breast cancer, such as family history.

According to NCI, several factors associated with alcohol use have been linked to cancer. Alcohol causes damage to DNA, which could lead to cancer development. Alcohol can also stop the breakdown of some nutrients that protect against cancers, including folate, carotenoids, and vitamins A, C, D, and E. Alcohol may also increase estrogen levels, leading to higher risk for breast cancer.

Tobacco

NCI reports that smoking causes an increased risk for numerous cancers, including lung, laryngeal, mouth, esophageal, throat, bladder, kidney, liver, stomach, pancreatic, colorectal, and cervical cancers, as well as acute leukemia. Smokeless tobacco products such as snuff and chewing tobacco increase the likelihood of cancers of the mouth, esophagus, and pancreas.

The 2004 Surgeon General's report on smoking cites previous reports regarding how our understanding of these risks has changed. One report noted a "significant association" between cigarette smoking and bladder cancer. However, a later reported stated, "Smoking is a cause of bladder cancer" and noted that quitting smoking reduced cancer risk in only a few years compared to people who continued to smoke.

In cancer of the voice box, or laryngeal cancer, the risk was known early on. The very first report from the Surgeon General in 1964 noted cigarette smoking to be a "significant factor in the causation of laryngeal cancer." They later upgraded this warning to say that smoking causes voice box cancer. Several other reports used similar language relating to oral cancer, going so far as to call cigarette smoking a "major cause" of oral cancer.

It should come as no surprise that the Surgeon General's reports note a relationship between cigarette smoking and lung cancer. Interestingly, a shift has occurred in the prevalence of certain types of lung cancer. Squamous cell lung cancer is on the decline, which seems to reflect the decrease in smoking overall. Lung adenocarcinoma is on the rise and is especially deadly to female smokers. Lung cancer death rates in men have been dropping. This shift in lung cancer rates can be linked to the decrease in smoking but may also be due to differences in the design of the cigarettes. Filters, vent holes, paper, and change in tobacco composition may be playing a part.

Part of this discussion in design change is the idea of the "light" cigarette. The trend of lower tar or light cigarettes has not created a safer cigarette. These cigarettes have not resulted in a decrease in cancer. In 2009, President Barack Obama signed the Family Smoking Prevention and Tobacco Control Act, which restricts tobacco manufacturers' use of the terms *light, low,* or *mild* to describe tobacco products. These terms are thought to confuse smokers into thinking these cigarettes are less dangerous than full-flavored cigarettes. Many of these varieties are still available, but without those words in the name.

According to NCI, tobacco smoke contains 7,000 chemicals, at least 250 of which are known to be harmful. Of those 250 chemicals, 69 are classified as carcinogens, including hydrogen cyanide, carbon monoxide, ammonia, arsenic, benzene, beryllium, cadmium, nickel, and formaldehyde. Any of these carcinogens can cause mutations resulting in cancer growth—either through direct contact with the smoke, such as in lung cancer, or through the bloodstream, such as in bladder cancer.

The Effect of Cessation

The research on cigarette smoking is clear: quitting smoking has a positive effect on health. See Figure 6-2 for a timeline of health improvements related to cancer and cardiovascular risk reduction over time. Even stopping at the time of a lung cancer diagnosis appears to be beneficial. Several researchers looked at early-stage lung cancer and quitting smoking at diagnosis. When smokers quit at diagnosis, they more than doubled their chance of survival over five years to 63%, versus a rate of 29% if they continued smoking. The increased survival chance results not just from reducing the progression of lung cancer, but also from the reduction of other smoking-related diseases such as COPD.

Figure 6-2. Benefits of Quitting Smoking

- 20 minutes after quitting: heart rate drops to normal.
- 12 hours: carbon monoxide level in the blood drops to normal.
- 2 weeks to 3 months: risk of heart attack drops; lung function begins to improve.
- 1–9 months: coughing and shortness of breath decrease.
- 1 year: risk of coronary heart disease is half that of a smoker.
- 5–15 years: stroke risk is reduced to that of a nonsmoker; risk of mouth, throat, and esophageal cancer is half that of a smoker.
- 10 years: risk of dying from lung or bladder cancer is half that of a smoker; risk of cervical, laryngeal, kidney, and pancreatic cancer is decreased.
- 15 years: risk of coronary heart disease is the same as that of a non-smoker.

Note. Based on information from U.S. Department of Health and Human Services, 2004.

 FACT OR FICTION: **Free tobacco cessation resources are available in every state.**

Fact. There are, indeed, free tobacco cessation resources in every state. Visit https://smokefree.gov to identify resources in your state or to sign up for effective cessation programs and find accurate information and professional cessation assistance.

Unfortunately, the data are less clear related to stopping alcohol consumption. IARC has studied the link between alcohol and cancer. For laryngeal cancer, study participants who smoked and drank derived benefit from smoking cessation, and the study noted a decrease in cancer rates, whereas nonsmokers who drank alcohol and quit did not see a decreased risk until 20 years after cessation. Laryngeal cancer rates in years 1–19 remained about 25% higher than for people who never drank alcohol. When looking at esophageal cancer, the benefit of alcohol cessation was not seen until about 10 years after quitting. Unfortunately, there is not a lot of additional information about the cancer risk reduction benefits of stopping drinking. Of course, we know that when heavy drinkers quit, they see immediate benefits of decreased risk of motor vehicle crashes, no hangovers, and no blackouts.

The Safe Amount of Alcohol and Tobacco

Alcohol

NIAAA has defined different levels of alcohol consumption and the standard drink sizes in the United States: 12 fluid ounces of beer (5% alcohol), 5 fluid ounces of wine (12% alcohol), or 1.5 fluid ounces of 80-proof liquor (40% alcohol). As a caveat, some beverages contain more alcohol than the standard. For example, some specialty beers have an alcohol content anywhere from 7%–12%. The same is true of certain wines. An alcohol's proof is essentially double the alcohol percentage. If a bottle of hard liquor is 100 proof, it is 50% alcohol. NIAAA further defines the amount of drinking with a low risk of developing an alcohol use disorder as *moderate drinking*. Women should drink no more than three drinks on any single day and no more than seven drinks in a week. Men should drink no more than four drinks in a single day and no more than 14 drinks per week. As you can see, by these rules, you can't "save up" your drinks and drink all 14 on a Saturday night. If you stay within these amounts or less, according to NIAAA, you have a 2% risk of developing an alcohol use disorder. The American Cancer Society recommends women limit themselves to one drink per day and men to no more than two drinks per day. These levels keep an individual below the threshold for increased risk for cancer. A word of warning: even drinking within these limits, you can have issues if other health problems exist or if you simply drink too quickly.

NIAAA suggests complete avoidance of alcohol in certain cases, including when driving a vehicle or operating machinery. People taking medications with a known interaction with alcohol should also avoid alcohol. Individuals with a medical condition that can be aggravated by alcohol should also avoid drinking. Finally, pregnant women and women trying to get pregnant should not drink.

Lastly, if you are thinking of adding wine or other alcoholic beverages to your heart-healthy diet, you may want to reconsider. Although some research suggests that wine and other alcohol may increase high-density lipoprotein, known as HDL (good) cholesterol, provide antioxidants, and promote anticlotting—all heart-healthy goals—the jury is still out on the benefits of alcohol consumption. The American Heart Association stops short of recommending any sort of alcohol regimen for heart health. They encourage people to talk to their healthcare providers about lowering cholesterol, lowering blood pressure, controlling weight, getting enough exercise, and eating a healthy diet.

Tobacco

No amount nor form of tobacco use is safe. Researchers have studied the effects of smoking just 1–4 cigarettes per day. Compared to never smokers, people who smoke 1–4 cigarettes have a 2.74 times greater risk of heart attack, with men having a 2.79 times greater lung cancer risk and women having a whopping 5 times higher lung cancer risk. The risk of death from all causes was about 50% higher for both men and women compared to never smokers.

No other form of smoking—cigar, hookah (water bowl), or other variations—is noted to be safer. Smokeless tobaccos such as snuff or chewing tobacco may not cause lung cancer, but the risk of oral cancer is substantial. Although they do not contain tobacco, electronic nicotine devices such as e-cigarettes or "vaping" have been under U.S. Food and Drug Administration control as a tobacco product since the fall of 2016.

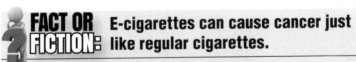

FACT OR FICTION: E-cigarettes can cause cancer just like regular cigarettes.

Unknown. Not enough information is currently known about this sort of nicotine delivery. Certainly, e-cigarettes have the cardiac side effects and addictive properties of nicotine. It is not known if nicotine alone is a carcinogen. Numerous studies are underway to research e-cigarettes and their suspected links to acute and chronic diseases.

Summary

Clearly, alcohol and especially tobacco present a serious health risk not only for the development of cancer but for other health problems as well. Figure 6-3 summarizes the cancers implicated for each of these drugs. Although you can achieve a middle ground for responsibly drinking alcohol, no degree of tobacco use is safe. If you already consume alcohol, to diminish health risks, you should decrease consumption to at least the level of a moderate drinker (as defined by NIAAA) or stop entirely. Individuals should not start drinking alcohol to derive heart health benefits because research on this subject is not conclusive. Healthcare providers can discuss safer alternatives and help develop a complete heart health strategy. When a person quits using tobacco, the benefits appear quickly, and the risks for many health problems decrease quickly, too. Even people already diagnosed with

Figure 6-3. Increased Cancer Risks From Alcohol and Tobacco

Alcohol	Tobacco
• Breast cancer	• Acute myeloid leukemia
• Colon cancer	• Bladder cancer
• Esophageal cancer	• Cervical cancer
• Laryngeal cancer	• Colorectal cancer
• Liver cancer	• Esophageal cancer
• Oral cavity cancer	• Kidney cancer
• Throat cancer	• Laryngeal cancer
	• Liver cancer
	• Lung cancer
	• Oral cavity cancer
	• Pancreatic cancer
	• Stomach cancer
	• Throat cancer

Note. Based on information from National Cancer Institute, 2013, 2017.

lung cancer can survive longer if they quit at the time of diagnosis, so it is never too late to quit.

Recommended Reading

American Cancer Society. (2015). Why people start smoking and why it's hard to stop. Retrieved from http://www.cancer.org/cancer/cancercauses /tobaccocancer/why-people-start-using-tobacco

Dudley, R. (2014). *The drunken monkey: Why we drink and abuse alcohol.* Berkeley, CA: University of California Press.

U.S. Department of Health and Human Services, Public Health Service, Office of the Surgeon General. (2014). *The health consequences of smoking—50 years of progress: A report of the Surgeon General.* Retrieved from http://www .surgeongeneral.gov/library/reports/50-years-of-progress/full-report.pdf

Glossary

cardiomyopathy [kahr-dee-oh-mahy-op-uh-thee]—Any disease of the heart muscle leading to decreased function; usually of unknown cause.

cirrhosis [si-roh-sis]—A disease of the liver characterized by increase of connective tissue and alteration in gross and microscopic makeup.

larynx [lar-ingks]—A muscular and cartilaginous structure lined with mucous membrane at the upper part of the trachea in humans, where the vocal cords are located.

CHAPTER 7

Viruses and Vaccines

Colleen H. Erb, MSN, CRNP, ACNP-BC, AOCNP®

Vaccines are the tugboats of preventive health.
—William Foege, MD, MPH,
developer of the global strategy that
eradicated smallpox in the 1970s

According to a 2016 *Lancet Global Health* study, 15.4% of the 14 million new global cancer cases in 2012 were associated with cancer-causing infections, including viruses, bacteria, and parasites. The study also found that cancer rates associated with infections are higher in developing countries. Less than 5% of new cancer cases in the United States, Canada, Australia, New Zealand, and some countries in western and northern Europe are associated with infections, compared to 50% or more of the cases in some countries in sub-Saharan Africa being associated with infections. Some, if not most, of these infections are preventable, and preventing them would decrease the overall rate of cancer, especially those involving the liver, cervix, genitals, and head and neck. The International Agency for Research on Cancer has classified 11 different bacteria, viruses, and parasites as cancer-causing infections in humans. In November 2016, the National Institutes of Health added seven substances to the *14th Report on Carcinogens*, of which five were viruses (see Figure 7-1).

This chapter will focus on those cancer-causing infections that can be prevented by vaccination, namely hepatitis B and human papillo-

---

Figure 7-1. Bacteria, Viruses, and Parasites Known to Cause Cancer in Humans

- *Helicobacter pylori* bacteria
- Hepatitis B virus
- Hepatitis C virus
- Human immunodeficiency virus type 1 (HIV-1)
- High-risk human papillomavirus
- Epstein-Barr virus
- Human herpesvirus type 8 (HHV-8 or Kaposi sarcoma herpesvirus)
- Human T-cell lymphotropic virus type 1 (HTLV-1)
- *Opisthorchis viverrini* parasite (Southeast Asian liver fluke)
- *Clonorchis sinensis* parasite (Chinese liver fluke)
- *Schistosoma haematobium* parasite, which causes schistosomiasis, known as snail fever (found in Africa and the Middle East)

Note. Based on information from National Toxicology Program, 2016.

---

mavirus, as well as a brief overview of new developments in the treatment of cancer using vaccines to stimulate the immune system.

FACT OR FICTION: Vaccines cause autism spectrum disorder.

Fiction. Numerous studies have looked at the suspected link between vaccination and the increase in autism spectrum disorder. To date, no study has identified vaccines as a cause of autism spectrum disorder.

Hepatitis B

Hepatitis B is a virus that causes serious liver disease either by acute or chronic infection. Acute infection is a short-term illness that usually appears within six months of exposure. Acute hepatitis B causes flu-like symptoms, including fever, fatigue, muscle or joint pain, and stomachache, but it can also be associated with jaundice (yellowing of the eyes or skin), dark urine, and clay-colored bowel movements. Chronic hepatitis B occurs when the virus remains in a person's body for a long period of time. Chronic infection may not have any symptoms, but it can lead to cirrhosis and is a leading cause of liver cancer. Chronic hepatitis B infection can also be linked to some types of non-Hodgkin lymphoma. (The hepatitis C virus can also lead to cirrhosis and liver cancer but as of now does not have a vaccine available.)

Impact of Hepatitis B

The World Health Organization (WHO) reported that approximately 240 million people globally have chronic hepatitis B infection, and more than 686,000 people die every year from complications of hepatitis B, including cirrhosis and liver cancer. Hepatitis B spreads through contact with the blood or body fluids of an infected person. The virus can survive outside the body for at least seven days, and during this time, the virus can still cause infection if it enters the body of a person not protected against the virus. The **incubation period** (the time between infection and showing symptoms) of hepatitis B is approximately 75 days, but it can be as little as 30 days and as much as 180 days. The virus can be detected within 30–60 days after a person has been exposed. WHO data indicate hepatitis B prevalence is highest in sub-Saharan Africa and East Asia, where as many as 5%–10% of the adult population is chronically infected. Higher rates of infection have been found in the Amazon region of South America and in southeast and south-central Europe. In the Middle East and India, approximately 2%–5% of the population has hepatitis B. In comparison, less than 1% of those living in Western Europe and North America are chronically infected. In children, 30%–50% of those infected before age six develop chronic infections. In adults, 20%–30% of those infected will develop cirrhosis or liver cancer.

Liver cancer arising from chronic hepatitis B infection can progress rapidly and has limited treatment options. The outcome for people with liver cancer from chronic hepatitis B infection is generally poor. In developing countries, people with liver cancer generally die within months of diagnosis. In more developed countries, surgery and chemotherapy can prolong life for a few years, and liver transplantation sometimes helps patients with only cirrhosis in these settings.

Vaccination

Vaccination can prevent hepatitis B, and a vaccine has been available since 1982. The hepatitis B vaccine is 95% effective in preventing infection and the development of chronic disease and liver cancer related to hepatitis B. The vaccine contains parts of the hepatitis B virus, but it cannot cause infection. The vaccine is given as three injections spread over a six-month period. In most cases, the vaccine is now given at birth and completed at six months of age; however, anyone who has not yet been vaccinated should be, especially those who work in healthcare settings, people working in public safety, and anyone who takes part in high-risk activities (see Figure 7-2). In 96 countries, hepatitis B vaccination is administered within 24 hours of birth. WHO reports that 38% of people worldwide are vaccinated, with a vaccination rate as high as 80% in the western Pacific but only 10% in Africa. Since the vaccine has been available, more than a bil-

---

Figure 7-2. People at High Risk for Contracting Hepatitis B

- People who frequently require blood or blood products
- People who require dialysis
- Recipients of solid organ transplantation
- People who are incarcerated
- People who inject drugs and who may share needles, syringes, or other drug injection equipment
- People who have household or sexual contacts with chronic hepatitis B infection
- People with multiple sexual partners
- Healthcare workers and others who may be exposed to blood and blood products through work
- Travelers who are planning to go to endemic areas
- Homosexual men
- Residents and staff of facilities for people with developmental disabilities
- People with chronic liver disease, kidney disease, HIV infection, or diabetes

Note. Based on information from Centers for Disease Control and Prevention, 2016b; World Health Organization, 2017.

lion doses have been administered worldwide. In many countries where historically 8%–15% of children were chronically infected, the introduction of the vaccine has led to chronic infection rates less than 1%.

FACT OR FICTION: Widespread hepatitis B vaccination has reduced cancer rates.

Fact. As of 2014, 184 countries have incorporated the hepatitis B vaccine into their national infant immunization programs, and vaccination has been shown to prevent liver cancer in children and young adults.

Vaccines can also have side effects. The side effects from hepatitis B vaccination are usually mild and go away on their own, but rare, serious reactions are also possible. Most people who receive the vaccine have no problems with it and do not experience any side effects. Minor problems after hepatitis B vaccine include soreness at the injection site and a mild fever of 99.9°F or higher for 24–48 hours. Although uncommon, fainting can occur. Sitting or lying down for 15 minutes can help prevent fainting and injuries caused by a fall. If people experience dizziness with medical procedures, have vision changes, or experience ringing in the ears, they should be especially cautious and be monitored for at least 15 minutes to prevent fainting. Some people experience more intense shoulder pain that lasts longer than usually occurs with an injection.

Any medication or vaccination can cause a severe allergic reaction. Vaccines very rarely cause this type of reaction, with an estimated one case of a severe reaction for every one million vaccines given. If signs of a severe allergic reaction occur after vaccination, including very high fever or unusual behavior, call your healthcare provider immediately. Signs of an allergic reaction can include hives, swelling of the face and throat, difficulty breathing, a fast heartbeat, dizziness, and weakness. Allergic reactions typically happen within a few minutes to a few hours after the vaccination.

In May 2016, the World Health Assembly adopted the *Global Health Sector Strategy on Viral Hepatitis, 2016–2021.* This plan highlights the critical need for universal health coverage and envisions eliminating viral hepatitis as a public health problem worldwide. Specifically, this plan seeks to reduce new viral hepatitis infections by 90% and to reduce deaths from viral hepatitis by 65% by 2030. Some of the strategies for this goal include raising awareness of the disease, mobilizing global resources, formulating evidence-based policies and data for action plans, preventing transmission with vaccination, and increasing screening, care, and treatment services.

Human Papillomavirus

Human papillomavirus (HPV) is a known cause of cervical cancer in addition to some cases of vulvar, vaginal, penile, head and neck, anal, and rectal cancers. HPV has 13 subtypes that cause cancer, and infection with any of these types leads to a much higher risk of cancer. A 2016 article published in *Morbidity and Mortality Weekly Report* reviewed five years of data and found that between 2008 and 2012, approximately 30,700 cases of cancer diagnosed per year were attributable to HPV, with men experiencing a much higher incidence of HPV-related cancers. Most cervical cancers are preventable with regular screening, treatment, and close follow-up for precancerous lesions in women aged 21–65. There are no routine screening strategies for the other HPV-associated cancers.

Effects of Human Papillomavirus

A person can contract HPV through skin-to-skin sexual contact with an infected individual, including vaginal, oral, and anal sex. HPV cannot be passed by casual contact such as shaking hands or hugging. According to the U.S. Advisory Committee on Immunization Practices, HPV is the most common sexually transmitted infection in the United States with approximately 14 million people newly infected every year. Most infections cause no symptoms and resolve on their own without any treatment, but persistent HPV infection can cause cervical cancer in women. It can also cause cancers of the genitals, rectum, anus, and head and neck, as well as genital warts in men and women. Most of the time, the immune system can fight off infection before HPV causes any health problems, but when the body does not fight off the infection, HPV leads to cancer and other health problems. More than 150 identified types of HPV exist, including approximately 40 types that infect the genital area. Genital HPV types are categorized according to their risk of causing cervical cancer. High-risk types can potentially cause cancer, while low-risk types can cause precancerous conditions, benign lesions, genital warts, or a disease called **respiratory papillomatosis**. The high-risk types—HPV16 and HPV18—cause approximately 70% of cervical cancer cases worldwide.

Vaccination

Currently, there are three approved vaccines to protect against HPV infection. Cervarix®, the HPV2 vaccine, or bivalent vaccine, is effective against HPV16 and HPV18, which cause many cervical, genital, anal, and rectal cancers. Gardasil®, the HPV4 vaccine, or quadrivalent vaccine, is effective against HPV16 and HPV18, as well as HPV6 and HPV11, virus subtypes that are known to cause 90% of genital warts. Gardasil®9, the newest vaccine, is effective against nine types of HPV: types 6, 11, 16, 18, 31, 33, 45, 52, and 58. These nine types of HPV are thought to cause the majority of all HPV-related diseases and cancers. Cervarix is 92.9% effective if administered according to protocol. In all studies, more than 99% of participants developed immunity to the virus about one month after completing the three-dose series for all three vaccines. HPV vaccination is recommended for preteen girls and boys so they are protected before exposure to the virus through sexual contact. The vaccine can be given as early as 9 years old and as late as 26 years old. As of October 2016, the Centers for Disease Control and Prevention (CDC) recommends that boys and girls younger than age 15 receive two doses of the vaccine, given six months apart. Children and young adults aged 15–26 who have not been vaccinated should be vaccinated with three doses. HPV vaccines produce a higher immune response if given to preteens rather than older adolescents. Administration of all three vaccines is the same. Each dose of the vaccine is injected into the muscle, preferably the upper arm. If given in two doses (for those aged 9–15), the second vaccine is given six months after the first. If given in three doses (for those aged 15–26), the second dose is given one to two months after the first dose, and the third dose is administered six months after the first. If the schedule is interrupted, it does not need to be restarted. The same vaccine type should be used for all three doses because no evidence exists concerning the effectiveness of the vaccination if the three vaccines are combined. Cervarix, Gardasil, and Gardasil 9 are not live vaccines and can be administered to individuals with weakened immune systems.

FACT OR FICTION: HPV vaccination increases promiscuity.

Fiction. To date, no studies or data indicate that young men and women who receive HPV vaccination engage in more high-risk sexual behavior compared to those who do not receive the vaccine.

HPV vaccines have been studied extensively, and during these studies, no serious safety concerns were noted. CDC reported some common, mild side effects, the most prevalent being pain at the injection site, which happens in approximately 92% of patients. Redness at the injection site happens approximately 48% of the time, and swelling at the injection site occurs in approximately 44% of people who receive the HPV vaccine. Other less common reactions include fever, fatigue, dizziness, nausea, headache, and joint or muscle pain. Fainting has been reported in adolescents and young adults receiving the vaccine (or any injection), and providers should observe patients for 15 minutes after administration of the vaccine to prevent fainting or any injury from falls. No evidence suggests the HPV vaccine causes fertility problems. However, people who do not receive the vaccine are more likely to become infected with HPV and develop HPV-related cancers. Treatment of cervical cancer related to high-risk HPV infection can include hysterectomy, chemotherapy, or radiation as treatments, which could leave women unable to have children. Treatment for precancerous lesions of the cervix can put women at risk for problems with the cervix, which can lead to preterm delivery or other issues during pregnancy.

Paying for Vaccines

As of the time of this writing, all Health Insurance Marketplace plans and most private insurance plans are required to cover several vaccines without charging a copayment if a network provider administers the vaccine (see Figure 7-3). Even if individuals have not met yearly deductibles, these vaccines should be covered by insurance. Medicare Part B will also pay for the hepatitis B vaccination for people who are at increased risk for contracting the virus. Medicaid agencies cover some, but not all, adult immunizations, and people covered by Medicaid insurance should check with their providers about coverage. TRICARE (military insurance) covers all vaccines recommended by the CDC vaccination schedule (see Figure 7-4), including hepatitis B. Insurances listed previously also provide HPV vaccinations, but uninsured individ-

---

Figure 7-3. Vaccinations Covered by Most Insurance Plans

- Hepatitis A
- Hepatitis B
- Herpes zoster (shingles)
- Human papillomavirus
- Influenza
- Measles, mumps, rubella
- Meningitis
- Pneumonia
- Tetanus, diphtheria, pertussis (whooping cough)
- Varicella (chickenpox)

Note. Based on information from Centers for Disease Control and Prevention, 2016a.

Figure 7-4. Recommended Immunization Schedule for Adults Aged 19 Years or Older by Age Group, United States, 2017

Vaccine*	19–21 years	22–26 years	27–59 years	60–64 years	≥ 65 years
Influenza	1 dose annually				
Td/Tdap	Substitute Tdap for Td once, then Td booster every 10 years				
MMR	1 or 2 doses depending on indication				
VAR	2 doses				
HZV				1 dose	
HPV–Female	3 doses				
HPV–Male	3 doses	3 doses			
PCV13	1 dose				1 dose
PPSV23	1 or 2 doses depending on indication				1 dose
HepA	2 or 3 doses depending on vaccine				
HepB	3 doses				
MenACWY or MPSV4	1 or more doses depending on indication				
MenB	2 or 3 doses depending on vaccine				
Hib	1 or 3 doses depending on indication				

* Please refer to the original source for important general information and considerations for special populations.

Hep—hepatitis; Hib—*Haemophilus influenzae* type b; HPV—human papillomavirus vaccination; HZV—herpes zoster vaccination; MenACWY—serogroups A, C, W, and Y meningococcal conjugate vaccine; MenB—serogroup B meningococcal vaccine; MMR—measles, mumps, and rubella; MPSV4—meningococcal polysaccharide serogroups A, C, W, and Y vaccine; PCV13—13-valent pneumococcal conjugate vaccine; PPSV23—23-valent pneumococcal polysaccharide vaccine; Td—tetanus and diphtheria toxoids; Tdap—tetanus and diphtheria toxoids and acellular pertussis; VAR—varicella

Note. Light shading indicates recommended for adults who meet the age requirement, lack documentation of vaccination, or lack evidence of past infection. Dark shading indicates recommended for adults with additional medical conditions or other indications. White indicates no recommendation.

From "Recommended Immunization Schedule for Adults Aged 19 Years or Older, United States, 2017," by Centers for Disease Control and Prevention, 2017. Retrieved from https://www.cdc.gov/vaccines/schedules/downloads/adult/adult-combined-schedule-bw.pdf.

uals can find help to pay for vaccines by visiting www.healthcare
.gov and learning about health coverage options or by going to
www.cdc.gov and searching for vaccine coverage. The Vaccines for
Children program provides vaccines for children aged 18 years
and younger who are uninsured, Medicaid-eligible, and American Indian or Alaska Native. More information about Vaccines for
Children is available at the CDC website.

Vaccines for Treatment of Cancer

Most people know that vaccines are used to prevent infections
that might lead to cancer, as presented in this chapter. These vaccines use a weakened or "dead" form of the virus or bacteria to
kick-start an immune response in the body and prevent infection by those same viruses and bacteria. Vaccines can also treat
cancer. These vaccines work similarly but do not prevent cancer
from forming; rather, they treat the cancer once it is diagnosed.
Vaccines prompt a person's immune system to mount an attack
against the cancer cells already present in the body with the goal
of destroying cancer cells or stopping tumor growth or spread. If
cancer cells remain in the body after other treatments, vaccines
can help the immune system kill the leftover cells. They can also
prevent cancer from returning after treatment. Cancer treatment
vaccines are a relatively nontoxic treatment.

Most cancer treatment vaccines are only available through clinical trials, which are research studies that involve volunteers with
a specific type of cancer. The only vaccine currently approved
for treatment is sipuleucel-T (Provenge®). This is a vaccine for
men with metastatic prostate cancer, which means the cancer
has spread from the prostate to other parts of the body and is
not responding to other therapies. This vaccine is customized
to each patient by using three steps. First, a healthcare provider
removes white blood cells, which help the body fight infections
and diseases, from the patient's bloodstream. Next, the provider
modifies the white blood cells in a laboratory to recognize and
target prostate cancer cells. The provider then returns the mod-

ified cells to the patient's bloodstream through a vein—similar to a blood transfusion. The modified cells use the patient's own immune system to find and destroy prostate cancer cells. This vaccine does not cure prostate cancer, but it has been shown to help extend patients' lives by several months compared with the other treatments available.

Currently, multiple other cancer treatment vaccines are in development and undergoing clinical trials (see Figure 7-5).

Figure 7-5. Cancers With Cancer Treatment Vaccine Clinical Trials Underway

- **Bladder cancer**—One study is testing the effectiveness of a vaccine made to contain HER2 cells that live on the surface of bladder cancer tumor cells.
- **Brain tumors**—Many studies are testing treatment vaccines aimed at certain molecules on the surface of brain tumor cells. Some focus on newly diagnosed brain cancer; others focus on cancer that has returned after initial treatment.
- **Breast cancer**—Studies are testing vaccines given alone and with other treatments, as well as preventive vaccines for those at high risk.
- **Cervical cancer**—Treatment vaccines are being tested; human papillomavirus vaccinations are approved for prevention of cervical cancer.
- **Colorectal cancer**—Vaccines that encourage the body to attack cells with antigens common to colorectal cancer are being developed; these antigens include carcinoembryonic antigen, MUC1, guanylyl cyclase C, and NY-ESO-1.
- **Kidney cancer**—Several vaccines to treat kidney cancer are being tested, as well as vaccines to prevent later-stage cancer from recurring. One vaccine is made from the patient's surgically removed tumor cells.
- **Leukemia**—Studies are looking at vaccines for several types of leukemia, including acute myeloid leukemia and chronic lymphocytic leukemia. Some are combined with other treatments, such as stem cell transplants, to help make those treatments more effective.
- **Lung cancer**—Several treatment vaccines are being developed to target specific antigens, including MAGE-3, found in 42% of lung cancers, and NY-ESO-1, found in 30% of lung cancers.
- **Melanoma**—Several vaccines are being tested for use individually or in combination therapy.
- **Myeloma**—Several trials are underway in patients who are near remission. Researchers are also testing vaccines for use in patients with **smoldering myeloma** and those who undergo an **autologous** stem cell transplant.
- **Pancreatic cancer**—Vaccines are being developed to boost the immune response to cancer cells to be used alone or in combination with other treatments.
- **Prostate cancer**—Researchers are trying to develop a vaccine for less advanced disease.

Note. Based on information from National Institutes of Health, 2017.

Because these trials change frequently, visit https://clinicaltrials .gov for a complete and up-to-date list. You can find active clinical trials that are taking volunteers by searching for a specific cancer type. If you have cancer, you can also discuss current, available clinical trials with your healthcare provider.

Summary

Infections from viruses, bacteria, and parasites cause a significant number of cancer cases globally. People in developing countries are at the greatest risk for various cancers resulting from infection, but these infections still affect people in developed countries. Hepatitis B and HPV particularly can be prevented through vaccination, and more research is underway to continue to prevent, as well as treat, cancers through vaccine administration.

Recommended Reading

American Cancer Society. (2016). Cancer vaccines. Retrieved from http:// www.cancer.org/treatment/treatments-and-side-effects/treatmenttypes /immunotherapy/immunotherapy-cancer-vaccines.html

Hale, D.F., Vreeland, T.J., & Peoples, G.E. (2016). Arming the immune system through vaccination to prevent cancer recurrence. *American Society of Clinical Oncology Education Book, 35*, e159–e167. doi:10.14694/EDBK_158946

Plummer, M., de Martel, C., Vignat, J., Ferlay, J., Bray, F., & Franceschi, S. (2016). Global burden of cancers attributable to infections in 2012: A synthetic analysis. *Lancet Global Health, 4*, e609–e616. doi:10.1016/S2214 -109X(16)30143-7

Viens, L.J., Henley, S.J., Watson, M., Markowitz, L.E., Thomas, C.C., Thompson, T.D., ... Saraiya, M. (2016). Human papillomavirus-associated cancers—United States, 2008–2012. *Morbidity and Mortality Weekly Report, 65*, 661–666. doi:10.15585/mmwr.mm6526a1

Glossary

autologous [aw-tol-uh-guhs]—From the same organism.

HER2—Abbreviation for *human epidermal growth factor receptor 2*. HER2 is a protein expressed by and involved in the growth of some cancer cells. For example, HER2 is overexpressed in 18%–20% of invasive breast cancers and affects the treatment as well as the prognosis of breast cancers.

incubation period—The time between exposure to a bacteria or virus and the showing of symptoms.

respiratory papillomatosis—Disease caused by HPV in which tumors grow in the air passages between the mouth and nose and the lungs.

smoldering myeloma—A very slow-growing type of myeloma in which abnormal plasma cells (a type of white blood cell) make too much of a single type of monoclonal antibody (a protein). This protein builds up in the blood or is passed in the urine. Patients with smoldering myeloma usually have no symptoms but need to be checked often for signs of progression to fully developed multiple myeloma.

CHAPTER 8

Physiologic Stress and Inflammation

Kelsey Haley, MSN, RN, OCN®

> *Dear Stress, let's break up. —Me*
> —Author unknown

To function properly, the body maintains a constant environment among all its systems. Physiologic stress occurs when the body faces a threat or demand, such as an allergen or toxin. This type of stress differs from psychological stress in that it involves the body's response to something physical, rather than mental or emotional. Usually, stress is a natural event that causes the immune system to launch an inflammatory response—a controlled, protective process that resolves a threat or demand and restores the body's environment for proper functioning. However, when this process begins or continues inappropriately, it may damage the body's cells and genetic material and lead to cancer. This chapter discusses the types of inflammation and the role of inflammation in cancer, as well as possible causes of and methods to limit inflammation.

Types of Inflammation

Generally, an inflammatory response is classified based on its characteristics and is considered either acute or chronic.

Acute Inflammation

Acute inflammation is a short-term process; it is the normal and protective form of inflammation. The acute inflammatory process begins when physiologic stress causes cells or tissues to release biochemicals that bring white blood cells to the site of damage. The white blood cells produce substances that cause cellular growth and division to repair any damaged tissues. Once the damages have been repaired, the inflammatory process ends.

Chronic Inflammation

Chronic inflammation is the abnormal, long-term, and potentially destructive form of inflammation. The acute inflammatory process becomes chronic if it continues after the source of stress has been resolved and the damaged cells have been repaired or if the inflammatory process fails to repair damage within a certain amount of time. Chronic inflammation may also be *idiopathic*, meaning it begins without a threat or demand.

The Role of Chronic Inflammation in Cancer

In the 1800s, pathologist Rudolf Virchow observed an increased presence of white blood cells within tumor tissues, suggesting that cancerous tumors develop from chronic inflammation. Over the years, multiple laboratory-, animal-, and population-based studies have confirmed Virchow's observations. Chronic inflammation plays a role in each of the three stages of cancer—**initiation**, promotion, and progression—which were discussed in Chapter 1.

Initiation of Cancer Due to Inflammation

As previously stated, acute inflammation is a controlled process that begins in response to physiologic stress and cellular damage. It ends when the source of stress has been removed and damages have been repaired. When this process continues too long or without reason, the ongoing collection of white blood cells and inflammatory products generates **reactive oxygen species** (ROS), a type of chemical that causes additional damage to a cell's genetic material, or DNA. These complex molecules contain the instructions needed for the body to grow, develop, and function. Unrepaired damage to a cell's DNA is referred to as a *mutation*. Although not all mutations are significant, some may lead to cancer.

Promotion of Cancer Due to Inflammation

After the initiation of a cancer-causing mutation, the next stage of cancer development is promotion. ROS begin to interfere with cellular communication, causing the inflammatory substances that normally encourage cellular growth and division to also support the growth and division of *mutated* cells when they fail to see the difference. This process results in increasing numbers of mutated cells and the promotion of cancer.

Progression of Cancer Due to Inflammation

As cancer develops, ROS activate cancer-promoting genes, called *oncogenes*, and inactivate cancer-controlling genes, known as *tumor suppressor genes*. These genes allow cancer to grow and invade other tissues, leading to metastasis.

Causes of Inflammation

The immune system generates an inflammatory response any time an outside factor causes stress and disturbs the body's environment. Such factors include allergens, toxins, infectious agents, and some health conditions.

Allergens

For some people, the body may see a medication, plant, food, or common substance as a threat and stimulate an inflammatory response. The amount of inflammation depends on a person's level of sensitivity. Common medication allergies include penicillin, sulfonamide-containing antibiotics, anticonvulsants, and chemotherapy drugs. Environmental allergens such as pollen, grasses, ragweed, and mold cause allergic reactions in many people. Inflammatory responses related to food are more common for foods that contain wheat, eggs, soy, milk, nuts, and shellfish. Other common allergens include pet dander, dust, latex, and materials found in plastics and cleaning products. Ongoing exposure to an allergen may result in chronic inflammation. Fortunately, visible symptoms of acute inflammation usually occur prior to the less visible symptoms of chronic inflammation, so people with allergies can take measures to avoid exposure.

Toxins

Many studies have found that frequent contact with various toxins forces the immune system to initiate the inflammatory response and the formation of ROS. Heavy metals, such as mercury and lead, hydrocarbons, pollutants, pesticides, tobacco, and alcohol may cause inflammation. Other chapters in this book discuss these substances in more detail.

Infectious Agents

As discussed in Chapter 7, viruses, bacteria, and parasites also pose a threat to the body and trigger the inflammatory response. Many of these infectious agents can increase the risk of cancer development by creating a chronically inflamed environment. Human papillomavirus, hepatitis B and C viruses, Epstein-Barr virus, HIV, human herpesvirus type 8, human T-cell lymphotropic virus type 1, and Merkel cell polyomavirus are associated with some cancers. The bacterium *Helicobacter pylori* infects the stomach and increases the risk of gastric cancer. Several studies suggest the bacterium *Chlamydia trachomatis*, known as the sexually transmitted infection chlamydia, may increase the risk of cervical cancer. The parasites *Opisthorchis viverrini*, *Clonorchis sinensis*, and *Schistosoma haematobium* may give rise to the development of cancer, as well.

Medical Conditions

Sometimes inflammation is the result of an abnormal immune reaction to normal tissues caused by a disease, disorder, or other health condition. Ongoing abnormal immune reactions are often referred to as *autoimmune diseases* or *disorders*. For example, inflammatory bowel diseases, including Crohn disease and ulcerative colitis, increase the risk of colon cancer. Metabolic or endocrine disorders, such as thyroid disease and diabetes, as well as obesity may also cause inflammation. Other autoimmune disorders associated with chronic inflammation, such as rheumatoid arthritis and systemic lupus erythematosus, may lead to certain cancers, including leukemia and lymphoma.

Methods to Limit Inflammation

Researchers have found that about 30% of all cancers are associated with chronic inflammation. Luckily, there are many ways to reduce and even prevent this harmful type of inflammation.

Limiting Inflammation Due to Allergens

If you have allergies to certain medications, plants, foods, or materials, it is important to inform your healthcare providers and others so you can avoid preventable exposures. If your allergies require medications or treatments, you should follow the prescribed remedies.

Limiting Inflammation Due to Toxins

You should also be aware of your exposure to heavy metals, pollutants, and other chemicals. The U.S. Environmental Protection Agency (EPA) sets standards for safe levels of heavy metals allowed in consumer products and homes, as well as public land and waters; monitors the levels of common pollutants; and evaluates the chemicals used in common products to ensure that the safest ingredients are used. In the event of exposure, you should follow EPA's recommendations regarding the specific toxin. Similarly, if you anticipate an exposure for some reason, you should adhere to the EPA guidelines and wear personal protective equipment, which refers to clothing, gloves, and safety goggles specifically designed to protect against hazardous materials.

Some occupations, such as those involving construction, farming, and manufacturing, may have an increased risk of exposure to heavy metals, pollutants, or toxic chemicals. Employers in these occupations must discuss this risk with their employees and follow the required safety precautions. Chapter 11 discusses hazardous substances in the workplace and home in more detail.

Limiting Inflammation Due to Infectious Agents

General health precautions, including handwashing and personal hygiene, may prevent infection, thus reducing the risk of inflammation caused by viruses, bacteria, or parasites. The exposure to some infectious agents may be prevented by practicing safe sex, limiting sexual partners, and avoiding IV drug use. As discussed in Chapter 7, vaccines are currently available to protect against human papillomavirus and hepatitis B. If you do contract an infectious agent, it should be treated with the appropriate antiviral, antimicrobial, or antiparasitic therapy.

Limiting Inflammation Due to Medical Conditions

Although not all inflammatory diseases increase the risk of cancer, if you do have a preexisting inflammatory condition, it is important to follow healthcare providers' recommendations on medication regimens and lifestyle changes, which may include dietary modifications.

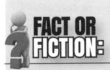 **FACT OR FICTION: People with inflammatory bowel disease have an increased risk of cancer.**

Fact. Both forms of inflammatory bowel disease, ulcerative colitis and Crohn disease, have been linked to colon cancer, and ulcerative colitis has been linked to pancreatic cancer in men. People with inflammatory bowel disease may need to have colonoscopies at an earlier age and more frequently. Individuals with these conditions should talk to their healthcare providers to learn more.

Limiting Inflammation in General

Antioxidants protect cells by preventing ROS from causing cellular damage. The body produces some antioxidants and obtains others from dietary sources. Vitamins A, C, and E, as well as beta-carotene and lycopene, are dietary antioxidants found in a variety of fruits and vegetables. Although some antioxidants are available as supplements, evidence has yet to confirm the value of such supplements in the prevention of cancer.

However, as discussed in Chapter 5, a diet high in fruits, vegetables, whole grains, and lean proteins that contain anti-inflammatory nutrients has been shown to reduce inflammation. Likewise, limiting dietary intake of pro-inflammatory nutrients, including refined sugars, polyunsaturated oils, and saturated fats, has been shown to lessen inflammation.

Regular physical activity, adequate sleep, and stress-reduction practices, such as yoga and meditation, improve overall health and may prevent inflammation. Additionally, avoiding tobacco and excessive alcohol consumption prevents unnecessary inflammation.

FACT OR FICTION? Daily use of anti-inflammatory drugs prevents cancer.

Unknown. Although anti-inflammatory medications, such as aspirin, ibuprofen, naproxen, and corticosteroids, reduce acute inflammation, research is underway to determine if regular use of these medications helps to reduce chronic inflammation and the risk of cancer development.

Summary

Although the immune system's inflammatory response is intended to minimize physiologic stress and promote cellular repair, it may react inappropriately in certain cases and result in cellular mutations that lead to cancer. Toxins, infections, and some health conditions can cause chronic inflammation, and a growing body of evidence supports a connection between long-term inflammation and cancer development. Fortunately, adopting healthy behaviors may reduce chronic inflammation.

Recommended Reading

Chai, E.Z.P., Siveen, K.S., Shanmugam, M.K., Arfuso, F., & Sethi, G. (2015). Analysis of the intricate relationship between chronic inflammation and cancer. *Biochemical Journal, 468*, 1–15. doi:10.1042/BJ20141337

Elinav, E., Nowarski, R., Thaiss, C.A., Hu, B., Jin, C., & Flavell, R.A. (2013). Inflammation-induced cancer: Crosstalk between tumours, immune cells and microorganisms. *Nature Reviews Cancer, 13*, 759–771. doi:10.1038/nrc3611

National Cancer Institute. (2014). Antioxidants and cancer prevention. Retrieved from http://www.cancer.gov/about-cancer/causes-prevention/risk/diet/antioxidants-fact-sheet

National Institutes of Health. (n.d.). *5 things you should know about stress* (NIH Publication No. OM 16-4310). Retrieved from https://www.nimh.nih.gov/health/publications/stress/index.shtml

Glossary

idiopathic [id-ee-uh-path-ik]—Of unknown cause, as a disease.

initiation—A process in which normal cells are changed so that they are able to form tumors.

reactive oxygen species—A type of unstable molecule that contains oxygen and that easily reacts with other molecules in a cell. A buildup of reactive oxygen species in cells may cause damage to DNA, RNA, and proteins, and may cause cell death. Reactive oxygen species are a type of free radicals, also called an oxygen radical. Abbreviated as ROS.

CHAPTER 9

Radiation Exposure

Kelsey Haley, MSN, RN, OCN®

Nothing in life is to be feared; it is only to be understood.
—Marie Curie,
discoverer of radioactivity

R adiation is the release of energy from a source. People are exposed to radiation daily from both natural and man-made sources. Researchers continue to study the relationship between radiation exposure and cancer. This chapter discusses the types and sources of radiation, as well as the role of radiation in cancer risk and methods to limit personal radiation exposure.

Types of Radiation

Radiation travels from a source in the form of energized particles or waves. The particles or waves are classified as *ionizing* (high-energy) or *nonionizing* (low-energy). The amount of energy, or radiation, absorbed by the body is referred to as a *dose*.

Ionizing Radiation

Ionizing radiation can damage DNA. Radon, x-rays, gamma rays, and ultraviolet (UV) light are common forms of ionizing radiation. Other forms of ionizing radiation include thoron gas, cosmic rays, and naturally occurring elements, such as uranium and radium.

Nonionizing Radiation

Nonionizing radiation does *not* have enough energy to damage DNA. Visible light and infrared are common forms of nonionizing radiation. Radiofrequency radiation and extremely low-frequency radiation are also forms of nonionizing radiation, but they carry less energy than visible light and infrared and are invisible. Sources of radiofrequency radiation include microwaves, radio waves, cellular phones, and radar. Creating, distributing, and using electricity are sources of extremely low-frequency radiation.

Sources of Ionizing Radiation

Radon

Radon is a colorless, odorless, radioactive gas released from the natural decay of rocks and soil. Depending on local land, this gas may dissolve into ground water or escape from the ground into the air, where it gives off radioactive particles. Outdoors, radon is quickly diluted to very low concentrations and usually not a concern. However, it may accumulate to higher concentrations in poorly ventilated areas and indoor environments, such as underground mines, caves, and water treatment facilities. Radon may even enter homes and buildings through cracks in the floors, walls, or foundation or from the building materials, such as concrete.

X-Rays and Gamma Rays

X-rays and gamma rays are forms of radiation that may be released by natural or man-made sources. Naturally, stars in space produce cosmic rays that release x-rays and gamma rays. The earth's atmosphere blocks most of these radiation sources, but some gamma rays and x-rays can reach the earth's surface.

Nuclear power plants generate man-made x-rays and gamma rays. The creation, testing, or use of atomic weapons may also release gamma rays and x-rays. Smaller doses of x-rays and gamma rays are used to perform various medical procedures, including radiographs, **computed tomography** (CT) scans, **positron-emission tomography** (PET) scans, and fluoroscopies, to detect problems of the skeletal system or diseases in soft tissues. Radiation therapy uses x-rays and gamma rays to treat or manage cancer. Additionally, x-rays and gamma rays are used to irradiate food to reduce bacteria, viruses, fungi, and insects known to cause foodborne illness or spoilage.

Ultraviolet Light

As discussed in Chapter 2, UV light is another form of radiation that is released by natural and man-made sources. UV rays have more energy than visible light but less than x-rays. They may penetrate the skin but not deeply into the body. Sunlight is the natural and main source of UV radiation.

Exposure to man-made or artificial sources of UV radiation can come from sunlamps, black lights, mercury-vapor lamps, and welding arcs. UV light is used in phototherapy to treat some skin conditions and may be used to kill bacteria and sanitize surfaces, water, air, or food.

The Role of Radiation in Cancer

As ionizing radiation passes through a cell in the body, it may damage the cell's DNA and cause a mutation. As a result of the mutation, the cell will either die or continue to replicate the mutation, leading to cancer.

The amount of damage caused in the cell and the risk of cancer related to radiation depend on the type and dose of radiation, as well as a person's age at the time of exposure, remaining life expectancy, and exposure to other carcinogens. Higher doses of ionizing radiation and greater exposure to other carcinogens, such as tobacco, have been associated with greater cell damage and cancer risk. Also, those exposed to ionizing radiation early in life and those with longer life expectancies have higher relative risks for cancer than others.

Cancer Risk Related to Radon

Studies of underground miners first confirmed that exposure to high levels of radon resulted in a greater risk of lung cancer.

Researchers analyzed several North American studies assessing the relationship between residential exposure to radon and lung cancer and discovered an increased risk of lung cancer associated with exposure to radon.

FACT OR FICTION: Radon is rarely linked to cancer.

Fiction. According to the U.S. Environmental Protection Agency (EPA), radon is the leading cause of lung cancer among nonsmokers and the second leading cause—behind smoking—of lung cancer among the general population.

Cancer Risk Related to X-Rays and Gamma Rays

The risk of cancer associated with the x-rays and gamma rays produced by cosmic rays has been studied, but no clear relationship has been found. Because these rays are present at the earth's outermost atmosphere, exposure is greater at higher altitudes. For example, people living in mountainous regions or traveling on an airplane have greater exposure than people at sea level or low elevation. EPA states that radiation from cosmic rays is low and unlikely to affect anyone's cancer risk.

However, the x-rays and gamma rays from nuclear plants and atomic bombs have been found to increase cancer risk. A notable study, known as the Life Span Study, examined survivors of the atomic bombings of Japan during World War II. This study is a major source of information regarding the health risks from exposure to ionizing radiation. The study first linked leukemia to the radiation exposure experienced by the survivors of the bombings. Leukemia is the most common cancer among these survivors. Later, other cancers were linked to radiation exposure from the atomic bombings, including cancers of the oral cavity, esophagus, stomach, colon, liver, lung, skin, breast, ovary, bladder, central nervous system, and thyroid.

Numerous studies have looked at the risk associated with receiving radiation for diagnostic reasons, such as radiographs, CT scans, and PET scans. The U.S. Food and Drug Administration estimates that exposure to one diagnostic test may increase the risk of death from cancer by 0.05%.

A more notable increase in the risk of cancer, especially leukemia, has been observed in those who received radiation therapy for the treatment of another cancer. The development of leukemia most often occurs within five to nine years after completing therapy. Radiation therapy may also increase the risk of developing some solid tumors, especially those of the breast, lung, and thyroid, depending on the location of therapy. These solid tumors usually develop 10–15 years after treatment.

It is important to know that while food irradiation does use x-rays and gamma rays to kill bacteria and other organisms, the food does not remain radioactive and does *not* expose an individual to radiation.

Cancer Risk Related to Ultraviolet Light

A clear relationship exists between the exposure to UV radiation and skin cancer. In fact, most skin cancers are a direct result of exposure to the UV rays in sunlight. In the United States, skin cancer is the most common cancer, and the number of cases continues to increase.

Methods to Limit Radiation Exposure

Exposure to ionizing radiation may occur in homes, public areas, workplaces, or medical settings. Although it is impossible to eliminate your exposure to all sources of ionizing radiation, you can reduce exposure to some sources.

Limiting Exposure to Radon

The amount of radon in the air is measured in **picocuries** per liter of air (pCi/L). The average amount of radon in the outdoor air is 0.4 pCi/L. The low concentration of radon in the outdoor environment is *not* dangerous.

FACT OR FICTION: Radon exposure is unavoidable.

Fact. Radon is a gas naturally produced from rocks and soil, so exposure to this gas is considered unavoidable.

The primary source of radon exposure for most people is in the home—through the water and air. The acceptable amount of radon in drinking water is 300–4,000 pCi/L; higher levels of radon are concerning and require intervention. A qualified radon professional can test a home's water supply, or you can purchase an at-home test kit online or at most hardware stores. The amount of radon in water is usually not a problem when surface water is the source. If water comes from the ground via a private well, an increased radon level is possible. Aeration systems or granular activated carbon filters are used to reduce high levels in drinking water.

Although a different method is used, a qualified radon professional or an at-home kit may also test the indoor level of radon in the air. A variety of kits exist, so it is important to follow the instructions provided by each kit. Short-term kits remain in the home for 2–90 days; long-term kits remain in the home for more than 90 days. The average indoor radon level is about 1.3 pCi/L. If an indoor environment has a radon level greater than 4 pCi/L, measures should be taken to reduce the level. With today's technology, the radon level of most indoor environments may be reduced to 2 pCi/L using measures such as sealing foundation cracks and openings, adding ventilation systems to increase air flow, and using pressurization systems to prevent radon from entering the home.

Miners, other underground workers, and those employed by uranium processing factories are exposed to greater doses of radon than the general population. The National Institute for Occupational Safety and Health (NIOSH) states that these workers cannot be exposed to more than 100 pCi/L within a seven-day period. NIOSH requires employers to inform employees about the risk of radon exposure, plan work to limit the amount of time spent in areas of high radon concentration, routinely monitor the levels of radon, use industrial fans to ventilate work areas, and provide respiratory protection.

Limiting Exposure to X-Rays and Gamma Rays

Environmental exposure to the x-rays and gamma rays produced by cosmic rays cannot be avoided, although the dose of these rays is low and unlikely to affect your health.

It is also unlikely that radiation from a nuclear power plant could harm the health of the general population. Today, nuclear power plants are highly regulated and safeguarded to protect the public from unnecessary radiation exposure. Choosing to live in regions far from nuclear power plants may reduce your risk of exposure to radiation in the unlikely event of a nuclear accident or disaster.

Approximately 80% of annual exposure to man-made ionizing radiation comes from medical tests and procedures. Although the increased risk of cancer from one medical test or procedure is very small, patients and healthcare professionals may reduce exposure by reviewing the necessity and usefulness of each test or procedure. Sometimes an alternative may be used that does not emit radiation, such as an ultrasound or magnetic resonance imaging (commonly referred to as MRI). If a radiographic study is necessary, shielding is used to protect parts of the body not being imaged from unnecessary radiation exposure.

Furthermore, if radiation therapy is determined to be the best treatment option for a cancer, the benefit of radiation outweighs the risk of developing a secondary cancer. Again, areas of the body that do not need radiation should be shielded. Once radiation therapy is complete, the patient should have follow-up appointments to monitor for secondary cancers caused by radiation treatment.

Occupations that involve exposure or potential exposure to x-rays and gamma rays should follow additional precautions. Such occupations include nuclear power plant workers, some military personnel, medical radiology and procedural personnel, and astronauts. The U.S. Nuclear Regulatory Commission inspects and provides licensure to users of radioactive materials and makes sure that radiation exposures are kept within specific dose limits and as low as possible. As with radon exposure, NIOSH requires employers to inform employees about the risk of radiation exposure and to use precautions to promote the safety and protection of their employees. Additional agencies set safety standards for specific occupations.

Limiting Exposure to Ultraviolet Light

Limiting your time in the sun and avoiding sunlamps and sunbeds lessens damage from UV light. The sunlight is especially harmful between mid-morning and late afternoon and at high altitudes. UV radiation from the sun is also reflected by sand, water, snow, and ice. When in the sunlight, you can reduce UV radiation exposure by wearing protective clothing, including long sleeves, long pants, a wide-brimmed hat, and sunglasses with lenses that absorb UV light. Additionally, sunscreen with SPF 15 or greater protects the skin from UV radiation, but its ability to do so is affected by proper use, sweat, water, and humidity. Sunscreen should be applied 20 minutes before sun exposure and reapplied at least every two hours.

Outdoor workers, including lifeguards, landscapers, and construction workers, should be diligent in limiting their exposure to sunlight and use sunscreen frequently. Welders and other workers that use UV radiation should use the appropriate safety precautions to limit their exposure, such as protective clothing, equipment, and filters. Employers must inform employees about the risk of radiation exposure and take measures to limit the potential of occupational exposure to radiation.

Summary

Expert organizations, such as the International Agency for Research on Cancer, the National Toxicology Program, and EPA, evaluate the likelihood of various exposures that cause cancer through laboratory, animal, and human research. According to these agencies, evidence exists to classify sources of ionizing radiation as carcinogenic to humans, including radon, x-rays, gamma rays, and UV rays. On the other hand, these agencies have found limited or inadequate evidence regarding the ability of nonionizing radiation sources to cause cancer.

The cancer risk associated with ionizing radiation depends on the type and dose of radiation and the age and lifestyle of the exposed individual. Although it is impossible to eliminate all sources of radiation exposure, it is important to take measures to reduce unnecessary exposure to radiation whenever possible.

Recommended Reading

Gale, R.P., & Hoffman, F.O. (2013). Communicating cancer risk from radiation exposures: Nuclear accidents, total body radiation and diagnostic procedures. *Bone Marrow Transplantation, 48*, 2–3. doi:10.1038/bmt.2012.90

U.S. Environmental Protection Agency. (2016). *A citizen's guide to radon: The guide to protecting yourself and your family from radon.* Retrieved from https://www.epa.gov/sites/production/files/2016-12/documents/2016_a_citizens_guide_to_radon.pdf

U.S. Nuclear Regulatory Commission. (2014). Minimize your exposure. Retrieved from http://www.nrc.gov/about-nrc/radiation/protects-you/protection-principles.html

Glossary

computed tomography—A sophisticated x-ray device used to obtain detailed images of internal organs. Abbreviated as CT.

picocurie—Unit measuring ionizing radiation; approximately the amount of radioactivity of 1 gram of radium-226. Abbreviated as pCi.

positron-emission tomography—A procedure in which a small amount of radioactive glucose (sugar) is injected into a vein, and a scanner is used to make detailed, computerized pictures of areas inside the body where the glucose is taken up. Because cancer cells often take up more glucose than normal cells, the pictures can be used to find cancer cells in the body. Abbreviated as PET.

CHAPTER 10

Genetics

Suzanne M. Mahon, RN, DNSc, AOCN®, AGN-BC

> *In your cells right now, an enzyme is making a copy of*
> *your DNA in less than two hours, right in the nucleus.*
> —Hugh Martin,
> 20th-century music composer

Approximately one in three Americans will be diagnosed with cancer at some point in his or her lifetime. Cancer occurs when normal cells begin to grow uncontrollably, forming a malignant tumor or an abundance of harmful cells. Most cases of cancer are not hereditary and can be prevented with a healthier lifestyle. Unfortunately, in about 10% of individuals diagnosed with cancer, the malignancy is the result of an inherited **mutation**—a harmful change in genetic material—that puts the individual at a much higher risk for developing cancer. This type of **gene** mutation can be passed down from generation to generation and often affects multiple members of a family. One of the most important things you can do to potentially reduce the chance of developing cancer is to know your family history and seek risk assessment and genetic counseling if many cases of cancer exist in your family.

Genes' Association to Inherited Cancer

Genes provide the instructions for normal cell growth and development. An error in a gene is called a *mutation*; some mutations prevent genes from functioning correctly. Acquired mutations (also called *sporadic* or *somatic mutations*) that occur after conception cause most forms of cancer. These cancers usually occur later in life because of exposure to cancer-causing substances over a lifetime. Mutations occur in one cell and are passed on to any new offspring cells. People with acquired mutations cannot pass them on to their children.

An inherited gene mutation is present in the egg or sperm that formed the individual. After the sperm fertilizes the egg, it creates one cell called a *zygote* that divides many times to create a human being. Because all the cells in the body come from this first cell, this kind of mutation exists in every cell of the body and can be passed to the next generation. This type of mutation is also called *germ-line* or *hereditary*. Inherited mutations are thought to be a direct cause in 5%–10% of all cancers.

Every human has 23 pairs of **chromosomes** that contain thousands of genes. We have two copies of every gene: one copy from our mother and one copy from our father. Most genetic changes that cause hereditary forms of cancer are inherited in an **autosomal dominant** manner, meaning the mutation only requires one parent to pass it on for the child to inherit the increased risk for developing cancer. Thus, it can be passed to a child by either the father or the mother. If an individual inherits a susceptibility gene from one parent, every cell in the body is affected with the mutated gene. Once the normal copy in one cell from the other parent becomes damaged from the environment or other exposure, the malignancy begins to develop. Because people with a hereditary cancer syndrome have a bad copy of the gene in every cell, they typically develop cancers more often than expected by chance and often at an early age.

Genetic testing is available to detect some harmful inherited mutations in families. Because each parent gives only one copy of each gene to a child, there is a 50% chance to pass the mutation to each child, male or female. Siblings of an individual with a mutation also have a 50% chance of having the same mutation if they share the same parent who carries the mutation. The risk for other family members to carry the same mutations depends on how closely they are related to an affected individual. It is important to remember that not all people who inherit a **pathogenic variant** in one of their genes will develop cancer; however, the risk does increase. See Table 10-1 for information on genetic syndromes and related cancers.

Table 10-1. Genetic Syndromes and Related Cancers		
Genetic Syndrome	**Genes**	**Related Cancer Types**
Hereditary breast and ovarian cancer syndrome	*BRCA1, BRCA2*	Female and male breast, ovarian, prostate, and pancreatic cancers
Li-Fraumeni syndrome	*TP53*	Breast cancer, soft tissue sarcoma, osteosarcoma (bone cancer), leukemia, brain tumors, and adrenocortical carcinoma
Cowden syndrome (PTEN hamartoma tumor syndrome)	*PTEN*	Breast, thyroid, and endometrial (uterine lining) cancers
Lynch syndrome (hereditary nonpolyposis colorectal cancer)	*MSH2, MLH1, MSH6, PMS2, EPCAM*	Colorectal, endometrial, ovarian, renal pelvis, pancreatic, small intestine, liver and biliary tract, stomach, brain, and breast cancers
Familial adenomatous polyposis	*APC*	Colorectal cancer, multiple nonmalignant colon polyps, and both noncancerous and cancerous tumors in the small intestine, brain, stomach, bone, skin, and other tissues
Hereditary retinoblastoma	*RB1*	Eye cancer (cancer of the retina), pinealoma (cancer of the pineal gland), osteosarcoma, melanoma, and soft tissue sarcoma
Von Hippel-Lindau syndrome	*VHL*	Kidney cancer and multiple noncancerous tumors, including **pheochromocytoma**

Genetics Professionals and Genetic Counseling

Genetics professionals are healthcare providers who have training, expertise, and certification in genetics and can manage genetic testing. They are trained to evaluate entire family histories and select the appropriate genetic test or tests. If a mutation is detected in a family, genetics professionals can arrange care for relatives who might benefit from testing and live in other geographic regions. Many insurance companies now require evaluation and counseling with a genetics professional before paying for testing. If you are concerned about having a genetic risk for developing cancer, consulting with a genetics professional is the best way to evaluate your risk. For a list of the types of professionals in genetics, see Figure 10-1.

These professionals provide genetic risk assessment services, family tree evaluation, and counseling before and after genetic tests. They also coordinate follow-up for other at-risk family members. An easy way to locate a genetics professional near you is to search online at www.nsgc.org.

Genetic counseling and testing can be extremely helpful for some families. Individuals who have a family history of cancer can start by speaking with their primary care providers about their cancer risk. Sometimes it is possible to estimate the chance of developing a particular cancer based on risk factors, such as a

---

Figure 10-1. Genetics Professionals

- **Medical geneticists** are physicians with board certification in genetics from the American Board of Medical Genetics and Genomics.
- **Licensed genetic counselors** are healthcare professionals with specialized graduate degrees in the areas of medical genetics and counseling who have been certified by the American Board of Genetic Counseling and have a CGC® (certified genetic counselor) credential.
- **Credentialed genetic nurses** have graduate degrees in nursing with specialized education and training in genetics and have received the AGN-BC (advanced genetics nursing, board certified) credential from the American Nurses Credentialing Center.

family history of cancer. When that risk is higher, sometimes a healthcare provider will recommend more frequent or intensive screening for that cancer. For people with multiple family members with cancer, a genetics professional can often help them to know if they need more intensive screening.

Some families have many cases of cancer, and some members may have a hereditary mutation that puts them at increased risk for developing cancer. A genetics professional can help a family decide if testing is appropriate, who is the best family member to test, and what might be the best tests to order. If an individual or healthcare provider is concerned about hereditary risk, a credentialed genetics provider can help a patient understand risks and discuss if genetic testing would be useful. Figure 10-2 identifies factors that could indicate families who may be at risk for hereditary cancer.

Healthcare providers and patients should consider these factors after gathering family history, and if one or more criteria are present, it may be wise to talk with a healthcare provider with expertise in cancer genetics.

Figure 10-2. Families Who Might Be at Risk for Hereditary Cancer

- A personal or family history of cancer at a young age (diagnosed prior to age 50)
- Two or more different cancers in an individual, either of the same type (such as breast cancer in both breasts or multiple colon cancers) or different types (such as breast and ovarian or colon and endometrial cancers)
- A pattern of cancer in which individuals with similar or related cancers are on one side of the family, spanning multiple generations
- Cancers occurring more frequently in a family than expected by chance in the absence of known environmental and lifestyle risk factors
- Presence of premalignant conditions, such as more than 20 colorectal adenomatous polyps
- Rare cancers, such as male breast cancer, triple-negative breast cancer, ovarian cancer, retinoblastoma, or pheochromocytoma
- People of **Ashkenazi** Jewish ancestry who have a personal or family history of breast, ovarian, or colon cancer
- Families who already have an identified mutation associated with increased risk for developing cancer

The Importance of Family History

The first step in genetic testing includes finding out how likely you are to develop a certain disease, as well as estimating your chance of having a mutation. This risk is based on medical history, lifestyle factors, and family history.

The genetics professional will ask many questions about your family. This important step provides extensive information so that the genetics professional can make the most accurate risk calculations and choose the best genetic tests, if appropriate. It is important to prepare for the appointment by gathering as much information as possible about the health of your **maternal** and **paternal** relatives.

During the first visit, the genetics professional will ask many questions about the health of your relatives, including discussion of children, siblings, parents, and maternal and paternal aunts, uncles, cousins, and grandparents. The genetics professional will want to know which relatives are alive and their ages, or if deceased, their age at death. The genetics professional will also collect information about any family member who has a cancer diagnosis, as well as other premalignant conditions, such as colon polyps. Because some ethnic groups are at higher risk for hereditary cancers, the genetics professional will ask questions about ancestry. The genetics professional will draw this information into a picture called a *pedigree* (see Figure 10-3).

The pedigree displays information about your family history in a visual format, and it sometimes makes it easier to see patterns of genetic transmission and possible genetic syndromes. Most genetics professionals will provide you with a copy of the pedigree if requested. The information in the pedigree also helps the genetics professional identify the best person or people to test first. If a test detects a mutation, the pedigree can be used to identify which other family members should be offered testing. Combined with genetic testing results, the pedigree provides information so the genetics professional can make the best recommendations possible for cancer prevention and detection.

Figure 10-3. Example of a Pedigree

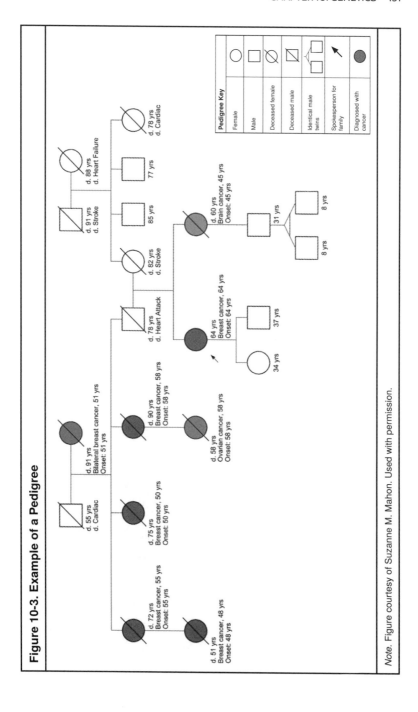

Note. Figure courtesy of Suzanne M. Mahon. Used with permission.

The pedigree should be reviewed at least annually and updated any time family history changes or the results of genetic testing become available for family members. Often, these updates will result in a revision of screening recommendations or additional testing for other family members. In some families, information on the pedigree is incomplete, which limits the accuracy of the pedigree. Sometimes family members are estranged or an individual does not have contact with an entire side of the family. Individuals who were adopted may have limited or no information about their genetic family history. The genetics professional will discuss how these problems affect genetic testing. Once a family realizes how important the pedigree can be for care, they will take the necessary steps to try to gather more accurate information.

Once the pedigree is complete, the genetics professional will evaluate it and discuss if any risks for cancer are increased. Sometimes genetic testing is not recommended, but more vigilant screening might be a good choice. Often the genetics professional will recommend some type of genetic testing. The decision whether to have genetic testing is based on information in the pedigree as well as personal risk factors. The accuracy of the pedigree determines the accuracy of the risk calculations and the selection of the genetic test.

Determining How Genetic Testing Is Ordered

Based primarily on personal and family history, the genetics professional will consider possible genetic diagnoses and suggest genetic testing. In the past, genetic testing has typically been focused on one or two genes. However, recent advances in genetics have identified many genes associated with hereditary risk. In most cases, genetic testing in a family now usually includes testing for multiple genes, which is called *panel testing*. A panel may be multiple genes associated with a particular cancer, such as breast or colon cancer. If the individual has had genetic testing in the past for one or two genes that did not identify a mutation, the genetics professional may suggest more expanded testing with a panel to identify a mutation.

FACT OR FICTION: If you're seeing a genetics professional, you only need to see that provider once.

Fiction. Genetics professionals recommend that individuals and families check back every 12–18 months to see if more testing has become available to identify a mutation and more frequently if family history changes.

If a mutation has never been identified in the family, the genetics professional will try to identify the best person to initiate testing in the family. Ideally, testing will be done in a family member who has been diagnosed with cancer—whether in active treatment or cured of the disease. Testing may provide helpful information for that person's care, as well as for other family members who do not have a diagnosis of cancer. A family member with early-onset disease, bilateral cancers (occurring in both of a pair of organs), or a history of multiple cancers is usually the best person to test. If an affected family member is not available for testing, testing of an unaffected family member can be performed, although a negative test result will not guarantee that the individual does not have an increased cancer risk. Once a mutation is identified in a family, other family members can usually have testing only for the specific identified mutation. Every family is different, and the genetics professional will help the family select the best test based on the family history. The science of genetics is ever changing, and families need to stay in contact with the genetics professional to receive the most current and comprehensive care available.

Considerations Before Having Genetic Testing

Once the genetics professional evaluates the pedigree and suggests that genetic testing is an option, a thorough discussion of the benefits, risks, and limitations of genetic testing takes place.

This discussion is a very important part of the genetic testing process (see Figure 10-4).

Figure 10-4. Activities That Occur During Pretesting Genetic Counseling

A genetics professional will
- Explain and discuss complex medical information about genetics and cancer.
- Explain how families inherit cancers and how genes are passed on to children.
- Describe the types of cancer seen in the family, and estimate a member's risk for developing these cancers.
- Discuss how genetic testing results might affect the person being testing, as well as how the results might affect other family members.
- Discuss the pros and cons, cost, and limitations of testing.
- Discuss who is the best family member to begin the testing process.
- Help each person make informed, independent decisions about health care.
- Assist the family with insurance preauthorization processes.
- Respect each person's individual beliefs, traditions, and feelings.

A genetics professional will not
- Tell a person which decision to make.
- Advise a couple not to have children.
- Recommend that a woman continue or end a pregnancy.
- Tell someone whether to undergo testing for a genetic disorder.

If you choose not to undergo genetic testing, you must have enough information to make a decision that is good for your individual situation. If you opt out of testing, the genetics professional will make recommendations for cancer prevention and early detection based on your personal and family history.

If you decide to undergo genetic testing, the genetics professional will have you sign a consent form prior to testing. The consent form acknowledges you have had the opportunity to explore the points outlined in Figure 10-5 and to ask questions. There are many things to consider prior to genetic testing, including the possible outcomes of testing and what genetic testing might mean for other family members. Education helps you prepare to deal with the possible consequences of test results. Other family members must decide whether

---

Figure 10-5. Components of Informed Consent for Genetic Testing

- Basic concepts of how genes work
- Purpose of the genetic test, a general description of the test, and the condition for which the testing is being performed
- Reason for offering the test and which people in the family are best to initiate testing
- Accuracy of the test
- Pros and cons of testing (including what the results might or might not tell you)
- What the test results mean, including positive and negative results, and the potential for uninformative results
- Screening options that could be used, depending on the test results
- Treatment options that might be available, depending on the test results
- Further decisions that may need to be made once the results are back
- Possible consent to use the results for research purposes after the test
- Availability of counseling and support services for the entire family
- Description of how the genetic testing is done
- Physical or emotional risks associated with the test
- Discussion of how the results might provide information about other family members' health, including the risk of developing a particular condition or the possibility of having affected children
- Plan for how and to whom test results will be reported and under what circumstances results will be disclosed
- Information about what will happen to the test specimen after the test is complete
- Statement that the person having testing has had the opportunity to discuss the test with a knowledgeable genetics professional
- Acknowledgment that the person being tested was informed that the alternative to testing is not testing and that the individual has the right to decline testing

---

testing is best for them or if they would prefer not knowing if they have a mutation. Because many considerations and consequences associated with genetic testing exist, pretest counseling is important in order to make an informed decision about what is best for you.

Genetic Testing Specimens

Genetic testing generally uses a specimen of blood or saliva depending on the test or panel of tests ordered. Results typically take three to four weeks to come back, sometimes longer. The genetics professional will discuss approximately when results will be available and how results will be disclosed.

Possible Genetic Testing Results

The results of genetic tests are not always straightforward and clear, which often makes interpreting and explaining them a challenge. Individuals and families need to be informed about the possible results prior to testing and have the opportunity to ask questions about the potential meaning of genetic testing. When interpreting test results, the genetics professional considers a person's medical history, family history, and the type of genetic test that was done.

Genetic testing can often help families better understand their risk for developing cancer. Testing is not perfect, so sometimes it is not possible to identify a mutation, but genetic testing can provide information to help many individuals and families make decisions about how to prevent or detect a cancer early. Genetic testing has three possible outcomes: positive, negative, and variant of unknown significance.

Positive Results

A *positive result* means the test identified a mutation that increases the risk for developing a certain cancer or cancers. Knowledge of having an increased cancer risk can assist in making medical management and treatment decisions with the goals of early detection and cancer prevention. In the case of a positive result, healthcare providers may make certain recommendations, such as the following:

- Starting screening earlier than usually recommended
- Screening more often than usually recommended
- Screening with tests that are used only for people known to be at increased risk
- Watching closely for signs or symptoms of cancer and getting any change promptly evaluated
- Learning about options to help reduce the risk of certain cancers, which might include medications or preventive surgery

- Adopting a healthier lifestyle, including smoking cessation, healthier eating, exercising, limiting alcohol consumption, and reducing exposure to ultraviolet light

Healthcare providers make these kinds of recommendations with the goal of preventing a cancer or finding it early when treatment is more effective.

Negative Results

Two types of negative results are possible. A *noninformative negative result* occurs when the first person tested in a family does not have a mutation. This result means the person tested negative for known mutations in whatever genes were tested. However, this result does not necessarily mean no hereditary risk exists. It might mean no hereditary risk is in the family, or it might mean some other mutation is present for which testing is not available.

For families in which members have a known mutation, a *true negative result* means the individual has not inherited the mutation. It does not mean no risk is present for developing cancer; it means the person has average risk and can follow regular recommendations for the prevention and early detection of cancer. A true negative result can help ease uncertainty and provide a sense of relief.

Variant of Unknown Significance

A *variant of unknown significance* means the test detected a change in the genetic material, but it is not clear if the change is a harmless or dangerous mutation. Sometimes there is not enough information about a genetic change—especially in "newer," more recently discovered genes—to classify it. To further clarify the clinical meaning of a variant, sometimes testing family members who have or had cancer may be helpful. If a relative with a related cancer has the same variant, it may provide evidence the variant is harmful. The more family members who carry the variant and develop cancer, the greater the likelihood the variant is harmful. If the variant continues to be found in family members with related cancers, in addition to other evidence, the variant may be reclassified as a mutation. At that time, genetic testing for the mutation can then be offered to other family members. In other situations, the variant is reclassified as harmless, and reclassification can often take years. Until a variant is reclassified, recommendations for cancer prevention and early detection are based on personal medical history and family history. Interpreting genetic test results can be complicated, and a genetics professional will explain what the results mean for the person tested.

Implications for Other Family Members

Typically, the first person tested in a family is tested for a panel of genes. If a test detects a mutation in the family, siblings, parents, children, and sometimes other relatives can be tested for that mutation. A genetics professional will identify which family members should be offered testing.

If a mutation has not been detected in the family or there is a variant of unknown significance, other family members might still be at increased risk for developing cancer, but testing will not be helpful—in the case of a variant of unknown significance— because it is not clear if the variant is a harmful or harmless change in the genetic material. In this case, the genetics professional will make recommendations for other family members based on their medical history and the family history of cancer.

Many emotions and unexpected consequences can surface when families learn the results of genetic testing. It can be frightening and upsetting to learn that you or someone in your family is at increased risk for developing cancer. Parents sometimes feel guilty or worry about passing the mutation to their children. Sometimes people feel relief even if they test positive because they can select a plan for cancer prevention and early detection that is more likely to be effective. Family members who test negative for a known mutation can feel relief that they did not inherit the risk and their offspring cannot inherit the mutation. However, they might feel guilty if other family members test positive. A genetics professional can help you and your family cope with these feelings.

Sometimes family members might not want to know if they may be at increased risk, especially if they can do little about it or don't want to undergo more drastic prevention measures, such as preventive surgery. Family members should know they have the option to test, but each family member must decide individually.

If a mutation is detected, it is the responsibility of the person tested to contact other family members and tell them they might be at risk and how to contact the genetics professional. Relaying this kind of sensitive information can be difficult, especially if family relationships are strained. Sometimes testing reveals family secrets, such as paternity, adoptions, or other difficult issues. Families need to realize that genetic testing can come with complications.

Clearly, genetic testing can be complex for many members of a family. Genetics professionals can assist family members in working through these issues and help each family member make the best decision for their individual situation. For these reasons, people who are considering genetic testing should speak with a genetics professional about these issues prior to testing.

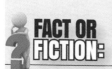

FACT OR FICTION: Genetic tests usually do not give a precise answer about inherited diseases.

Fact. Testing can only tell you if you have a specific gene mutation, not if you will get cancer. A positive test result does not always mean you will get the disease. The test can tell what might happen, but it cannot tell what will happen or when it might happen.

Limitations of Genetic Testing

A true negative result in a family with a known mutation does not mean there is no risk of cancer. The risk remains that of an average person, and risk can change over time because of lifestyle choices and simply getting older.

Some cancers may have only limited preventive or early detection measures. This can be unsettling and lead to anxiety. On the other hand, some cancers may have several ways to manage risk, and individuals may find it stressful to decide which to choose.

It is also important to realize recommendations for prevention and early detection may change. This could occur if a genetic variant is reclassified as a mutation, which can also occur as research reveals more about mutations. Also, newer methods of cancer prevention and early detection may become available. Genetics professionals can help individuals understand options and coordinate care with other healthcare providers. They are also a great source of information on new research. Sometimes, for families in which a mutation has not been detected, more testing could become available. Because the field of genetics changes rapidly, people who have undergone genetic testing or counseling should check back with their genetics professional, at least by phone, about once each year to see if the recommendations are still appropriate or if they need to be changed.

After Genetic Testing

Ideally, a genetics professional provides the results in person, but sometimes patients choose to receive results by phone or perhaps through video conferencing. Along with a copy of the results, the genetics professional also usually writes a letter that summarizes what the findings mean for the patient, what other family members should do, and specific recommendations for cancer prevention and early detection. The patient can share these materials with other healthcare providers.

The genetics professional will also help coordinate care for the rest of the family and can assist with finding a genetics professional located near other family members. The genetics professional can also guide you on how to reach out to other members in your family. Genetic testing requires long-term follow-up to ensure the best care possible for both the patient and family.

Insurance and Costs Associated With Genetic Testing

Genetic testing and counseling can have many associated costs. Costs and insurance coverage for genetic counseling can vary. When making an appointment for counseling, ask about the costs, and speak with your insurance provider about coverage.

The cost of the genetic testing itself can range from about $300 for a single-site test to more than $6,000 for a panel with many genes. The genetics professional can assist with obtaining insurance approval, and most laboratories will preauthorize the costs of testing. If there are out-of-pocket costs, many laboratories will contact the patient first to work out payment methods. The genetics professional will tell you the policy of the laboratory prior to sending a specimen. Many insurance companies, including Medicare and Medicaid, have specific criteria and prior-authorization requirements for genetic testing as a covered benefit. The genetics professional will explain whether these criteria are met and what it means in terms of coverage for the costs of testing. Concerns about the costs of genetic testing are very real, and the genetics professional will work with the laboratory and insurance company to try to make genetic testing and counseling affordable.

Discrimination Based on Genetic Test Results

The Genetic Information Nondiscrimination Act of 2008, also referred to as GINA, is a federal law that protects most Americans from discrimination by health insurance companies and employers with more than 15 employees. It does not apply to military health plans, the Veterans Health Administration, or the Indian Health Service. This law prohibits health insurers from using genetic information when deciding who to cover and how much to charge for insurance. GINA prohibits employers from discriminating on the basis of genetic information in hiring, firing or layoffs, pay, or other personnel actions such as promotions, classifications, or assignments. The law applies no matter how the employers obtain the genetic information.

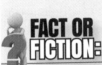

FACT OR FICTION: **GINA protects people from all potential forms of genetic discrimination.**

Fiction. GINA does not restrict use of genetic information for life insurance, disability insurance, or long-term care insurance. If individuals want more life, disability, or long-term care insurance, they should obtain this insurance prior to undergoing genetic testing. Prior to testing, the genetics professional will review the protections against genetic discrimination and possible risks of discrimination so the individual can make an informed decision about genetic testing.

Direct-to-Consumer Testing

Traditionally, genetic tests have been available only through healthcare providers such as genetics professionals. These providers are educated on how to order the appropriate test from a laboratory, collect and send the samples, and interpret the test results. *Direct-to-consumer genetic testing* refers to genetic tests that are marketed directly to the public via TV commercials, print ads, or the Internet. This form of testing provides access to a person's genetic information without necessarily involving a healthcare provider, genetics professional, or insurance company in the process.

If you choose to purchase a genetic test directly, the test kit is mailed to you, rather than to your provider. The test typically involves collecting a DNA sample at home, often by swabbing the inside of your cheek, and mailing the sample back to the laboratory. You are notified of your results by mail, over the telephone, or via the Internet. In some cases, a genetic counselor or other healthcare provider is available to explain the results and answer questions. The price for this type of at-home genetic testing ranges from several hundred dollars to more than a thousand.

At-home genetic tests, however, have significant risks and limitations. The results of unproven or invalid tests can be misleading. Without guidance from a credentialed genetics professional, you may make important decisions about treatment or prevention based on inaccurate, incomplete, or misunderstood information. Genetic testing provides only one piece of information about a person's health. Other genetic and environmental factors, lifestyle choices, and family medical history also affect a person's risk of developing many disorders. A genetics professional discusses factors during counseling, but in many cases, at-home genetic tests do not address these issues. Further, at-home genetic tests do not offer comprehensive evaluation for hereditary cancer syndromes; most only test for a few areas on some of the hereditary cancer susceptibility genes. This type of testing will fail to identify many of the hereditary cancer genes. If you are concerned about hereditary risk for developing cancer and are considering genetic testing, your best option is to get it with counseling and ordered from a reputable laboratory following discussion with a credentialed genetics professional.

Reputable Resources

Genetic testing for increased risk of developing cancer can be very complicated. Prior to testing, it is important to understand the implications and benefits of testing, as well as the possible risks and limitations of genetic testing. Social media and the Internet are filled with stories about genetic testing. Some of this information is reliable, and some is not. Reliable resources for more information are available in Appendix A. Genetics professionals can also suggest other reputable resources if you want more information.

Summary

Cancer risk assessment and genetic testing can be powerful tools to prevent cancer. The process begins with an awareness of how personal risk factors and family history affect cancer risk. Knowledge about cancer risk, especially in families with known genetic risk, enables the selection of the best possible recommendations for cancer prevention and early detection. Genetic testing is not just about one family member; the results of testing have implications for the entire family. Genetic testing can be confusing, and families often need assistance understanding the meaning of the results. Genetic counseling before and after testing is vital to help individuals and families understand the results of genetic testing when they first receive them and over time as risks change. If you or your family is concerned about hereditary risk, you should discuss these concerns with a credentialed genetics professional.

Recommended Reading

Lister Hill National Center for Biomedical Communications. (2017). *Help me understand genetics*. Retrieved from https://ghr.nlm.nih.gov/primer

MedlinePlus. (2017). Genetic counseling. Retrieved from https://medlineplus.gov/geneticcounseling.html

National Genetics and Genomics Education Centre. (n.d.). Telling stories: Understanding real life genetics. Retrieved from http://www.tellingstories.nhs.uk

National Society of Genetic Counselors. (n.d.). About genetic counselors. Retrieved from https://www.nsgc.org/page/aboutgeneticcounselors

Glossary

Ashkenazi [ahsh-kuh-nah-zee]—Jews of central and eastern Europe or their descendants, distinguished from the Sephardim (Jews of Spain, Portugal, and North African countries) chiefly by their liturgy, religious customs, and pronunciation of Hebrew. They are at an increased risk of hereditary cancers.

autosomal dominant [aw-tuh-sohm-ahl]—A pattern of inheritance in which an affected individual has one copy of a mutant gene and one normal gene on a pair of autosomal chromosomes. (In contrast, autosomal recessive diseases require that the individual have two copies of the mutation.) Individuals with autosomal dominant diseases have a 50% chance of passing on the mutant gene, and therefore the disorder, to each of their children.

BRCA—Either of two genes (*BRCA1* or *BRCA2*) that, if inherited in a mutated form, may predispose some carriers to develop breast or ovarian cancer.

chromosome [kroh-muh-sohm]—Thread-like structures in each cell that contain a person's DNA and genetic information. Humans have 23 pairs of chromosomes.

gene [jeen]—Basic unit of hereditary material that is passed from a parent to offspring and determines some characteristics of the offspring; a segment of a chromosome.

maternal—Having to do with the mother, coming from the mother, or related through the mother.

mutation [myoo-tay-shuhn]—A change in the structure of a gene, resulting in an altered form of the gene that may be passed to future generations. It can be caused by a change of a single base unit in DNA, or the deletion, insertion, or rearrangement of larger sections of a gene.

panel testing—A diagnosis-related group of laboratory tests.

paternal—Having to do with the father, coming from the father, or related through the father.

pathogenic variant [pa-thoh-jeh-nik vayr-ee-unt]—A genetic alteration that increases an individual's susceptibility or predisposition to a certain disease or disorder. When such a variant (or mutation) is inherited, development of symptoms is more likely but not certain. Also called deleterious mutation, disease-causing mutation, predisposing mutation, and susceptibility gene.

pedigree—A visual illustration of family history.

pheochromocytoma [fee-oh-kroh-moh-sy-toh-muh]—Tumor that forms in the center of the adrenal gland (gland located above the kidney) that causes it to make too much adrenaline. Pheochromocytomas are usually benign (noncancerous) but can cause high blood pressure, pounding headaches, heart palpitations, flushing of the face, and nausea and vomiting.

zygote [zahy-goht]—The cell formed when an egg and a sperm combine to make a fertilized egg.

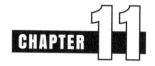
Cancer and the Environment

Tiffiny Jackson, RN, MS, FNP-BC, Tina Henderson, MPH, CHSP, and Stella Dike, MSN, RN, OCN®

> *The environment is everything that isn't me.*
> —Albert Einstein

Cancer is the result of changes in cell production, and often our environment causes these changes. *Environment* is most simply defined as the surroundings or conditions in which an organism lives or operates. This includes the air we breathe, the water we drink, the food we eat, and the places where we live and work. All can be potential contributors to the occurrence of cancer. There is almost daily discussion about possible relationships between our environment and cancer. Understanding the strength of those relationships—ranging from cell phone use (for which *no* conclusive evidence exists of a relationship) to sun exposure (for which a strong association with cancer occurrence *does* exist)—is essential to affecting how we engage with our environment. We must then scientifically evaluate the strength of these relationships based on documented evidence. This information can help us make healthy choices about potential exposure to cancer-causing agents.

This chapter addresses environmental concerns in homes, workplaces, and communities. The following information will identify which elements and exposures may play a role in cancer development and address popular myths around cancer and the environment. The purpose of this chapter is to help you identify which environmental factors to avoid when possible, which ones may be safe in moderation, and which ones do not have any scientific evidence of a connection with cancer.

A recent article in the *Annual Review of Public Health* identified tobacco, alcohol, ionizing and solar radiation, occupations, infectious agents, obesity, and lack of physical activity as accounting for nearly 60% of cancer deaths. Of these environmental factors, some are within our control, such as diet, exercise, and alcohol and tobacco use. Yet others, including exposure to radiation, viruses, and chemicals, are out of our control. The National Toxicology Program has identified 56 known (see Figure 11-1) and 187 "reasonably anticipated" carcinogens. These environmental factors work separately from, but sometimes with, genetic risks to influence cancer occurrence. Although all people face these environmental risks, exposure to carcinogens can harm children the most. How then should we interact with our environment to reduce these risks, especially given that some exposures are beyond our control? It is first important to understand existing environmental relationships in the United States and around the world.

Cancer in the United States

Approximately two-thirds of all cancer cases in the United States may be related to environmental factors, including diet and amount of exercise. Funding for studies of environmental contributors to cancer occurrence in the United States has been significantly limited, yet cancer trends suggest potential relationships between environmental carcinogens and cancer rates and mortalities. Cancer death rates are highest in Appalachia and Southern states and lowest in the Mountain states. Trends in cancer rates and death most closely relate to smoking and obesity—reflected by high overall cancer rates in areas with higher tobacco production, smoking prevalence, and fewer active tobacco control programs. Figures 11-2

Figure 11-1. Known Human Carcinogens

Substances Found Primarily in the Home
- Aflatoxins—produced by molds found in food
- Alcoholic beverages
- Aristolochic acids—plant-based compound found in some herbal medicines
- Azathioprine—immunosuppressive drug
- Estrogens, steroidal—hormones taken for a variety of health conditions
- Cyclosporine A—immunosuppressant drug
- Methoxsalen—compound used to treat skin conditions
- Mineral oils, untreated and mildly treated—substance present in lotions, creams, and ointments
- Sunlamps or sunbeds—devices used for self-tanning

Substances Found Primarily in the Workplace
- Chemotherapy agents used for cancer treatment
  - Busulfan
  - Chlorambucil
  - Cyclophosphamide
  - Melphalan
  - Semustine
  - Tamoxifen
  - Thiotepa
- Bis(chloromethyl) ether and technical-grade chloromethyl methyl ether—compound primarily present in the manufacturing of plastics, resins, and polymers
- Nickel compounds—present in industrial settings for the manufacture of products, including stainless steel and batteries
- Silica, crystalline—substance primarily produced through the chipping, sanding, and jack-hammering of substances such as granite containing silica
- Strong inorganic acid mists containing sulfuric acid—compound by-product primarily generated through oil refining and laboratory testing

Substances Found Primarily in the Community
- Benzene—organic chemical compound in crude oils and petrochemicals
- Coal tars and coal-tar pitches—substances present in asphalt products
- Coke oven emissions—generated during the heating of coal to produce coke for iron and steel manufacturing
- Erionite—mineral present in volcanic ash
- 1,3-Butadiene—chemical in motor vehicle emissions
- Ultraviolet radiation given off by the sun

Substances Present Across Settings
- Arsenic—an inorganic compound found in alloys and potentially water sources
- Asbestos—fibers present in insulation and other building materials
- Beryllium and beryllium compounds—inorganic compounds used for thermal conductivity in semiconductors and other devices
- Cadmium and cadmium compounds—metal found primarily in NiCad batteries

(Continued on next page)

Figure 11-1. Known Human Carcinogens *(Continued)*

Substances Present Across Settings *(cont.)*
- Chromium hexavalent compounds—used primarily in the steel industry in the production of alloys, stainless steel, and heat-resisting steel
- Ethylene oxide—chemical compound present in detergents, solvents, plastics, and disinfectants
- Formaldehyde—organic compound present in diverse substances, including resins
- Hepatitis B virus, hepatitis C virus—viruses affecting the liver
- Human papillomavirus—virus transmitted through prolonged skin-to-skin contact
- Radon—chemical element present as an airborne molecule
- Soot—carbon particles resulting from gas-phase combustion
- Tobacco smoke, smokeless tobacco, secondhand smoke
- 2-Naphthylamine—chemical compound found in cigarette smoke

Substances With Limited or Discontinued Manufacture Due to Carcinogenic Properties
- Analgesic mixtures containing phenacetin—fever-reducing medication
- Benzidine—chemical used to produce dyes
- Diethylstilbestrol—synthetic, nonsteroidal estrogen no longer produced in the United States
- Dyes metabolized to benzidine—chemicals used for dye production
- 4-Aminobiphenyl—chemical used primarily in laboratory settings
- Mustard gas—chemical compound primarily used as a chemical warfare agent but also for certain cancer therapies
- Thorium dioxide—radioactive chemical compound that may be used in nuclear reactors
- 2,3,7,8-Tetrachlorodibenzo-p-dioxin—chemical compound primarily used for research and may be produced as a side product of herbicides

---

through 11-4 represent the Centers for Disease Control and Prevention's trends in tobacco use, cancer rates, and cancer death.

States such as Kentucky and West Virginia demonstrate some of the highest rates of smoking, cancer incidence, and cancer mortality. However, death rates are consistently higher in Southern states despite cancer rates being higher in other parts of the country. Ultimately, environmentally linked cancer trends in the United States are largely based on behavior, not linked to chemicals.

Figure 11-2. Tobacco Use in the United States

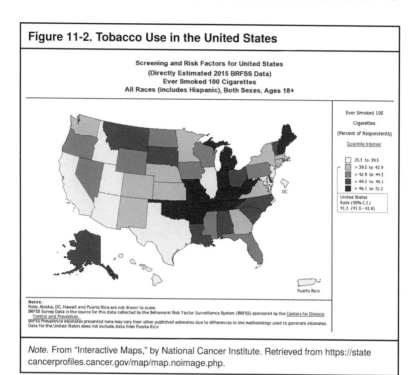

Screening and Risk Factors for United States
(Directly Estimated 2015 BRFSS Data)
Ever Smoked 100 Cigarettes
All Races (includes Hispanic), Both Sexes, Ages 18+

Ever Smoked 100
Cigarettes
(Percent of Respondents)

Quantile Interval

- 25.3 to 39.5
- > 39.5 to 42.9
- > 42.9 to 44.2
- > 44.2 to 46.1
- > 46.1 to 51.2

United States
Rate (95% C.I.)
41.3 (41.0 - 41.6)

Puerto Rico

Notes:
Note: Alaska, DC, Hawaii and Puerto Rico are not drawn to scale.
BRFSS Survey Data is the source for this data collected by the Behavioral Risk Factor Surveillance System (BRFSS) sponsored by the Centers for Disease Control and Prevention.
BRFSS Prevalence estimates presented here may vary from other published estimates due to differences in the methodology used to generate estimates.
Data for the United States does not include data from Puerto Rico

Note. From "Interactive Maps," by National Cancer Institute. Retrieved from https://state cancerprofiles.cancer.gov/map/map.noimage.php.

Global Cancer Trends

A 2015 study in *Cancer Epidemiology, Biomarkers and Prevention* indicates cancer is one of the leading causes of death worldwide, accounting for 8.2 million deaths in 2012, as well as 14.1 million new cases. The World Health Organization indicates environmental exposure plays a significant role in the incidence of cancer, accounting for 19% of all cancers and 1.3 million deaths. As in the United States, global cancer risk is associated with tobacco use, diet, and activity level. These risks are specifically reflected in recent increases in breast, lung, and colon cancers in developing countries. Furthermore, cancers related to infectious agents occur more often in developing countries, affecting the cervix, liver, and stomach. Connections between environmental pollution and lung cancer have been identified in several studies, in addition to increased risk from tobacco use.

Figure 11-3. Cancer Incidence in the United States (All Disease Sites)

Incidence Rates† for United States
All Cancer Sites, 2014
All Races (includes Hispanic), Both Sexes, All Ages

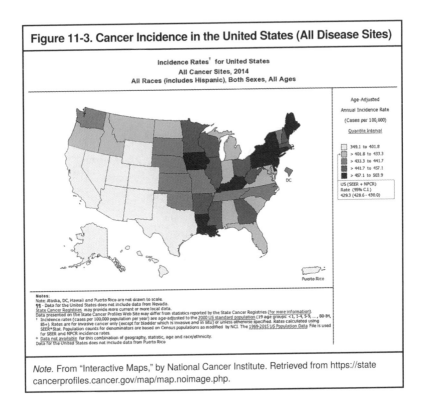

Age-Adjusted
Annual Incidence Rate
(Cases per 100,000)
Quantile Interval

349.1 to 401.8
> 401.8 to 433.3
> 433.3 to 441.7
> 441.7 to 457.1
> 457.1 to 503.9

US (SEER + NPCR)
Rate (95% C.I.)
429.3 (428.6 - 430.0)

DC

Puerto Rico

Notes:
Note: Alaska, DC, Hawaii and Puerto Rico are not drawn to scale.
¶¶ - Data for the United States does not include data from Nevada.
State Cancer Registries may provide more current or more local data.
Data presented on the State Cancer Profiles Web Site may differ from statistics reported by the State Cancer Registries (for more information).
† Incidence rates (cases per 100,000 population per year) are age-adjusted to the 2000 US standard population (19 age groups: <1, 1-4, 5-9, ... , 80-84, 85+). Rates are for invasive cancer only (except for bladder which is invasive and in situ) or unless otherwise specified. Rates calculated using SEER*Stat. Population counts for denominators are based on Census populations as modified by NCI. The 1969-2015 US Population Data File is used for SEER and NPCR incidence rates.
◊ Data not available for this combination of geography, statistic, age and race/ethnicity.
Data for the United States does not include data from Puerto Rico

Note. From "Interactive Maps," by National Cancer Institute. Retrieved from https://state cancerprofiles.cancer.gov/map/map.noimage.php.

The National Cancer Institute reported the second most common cause of lung cancer death in the United States is from air pollution, accounting for 223,000 lung cancer deaths in 2010. The World Health Organization estimated about 108,000 of the total lung cancer deaths globally each year are associated with outdoor air pollution, 36,000 are from solid fuels for indoor cooking and heating, and 21,000 are from secondhand smoke. Exposure to ambient (fine particle) air pollution has been associated with 16% of lung cancer deaths. Despite efforts to reduce global air pollution, it increased by 8% from 2008 to 2013, with the highest rates occurring in low- and middle-income countries.

In addition to lung cancer, other global cancer concerns exist related to the environment. For example, ultraviolet light expo-

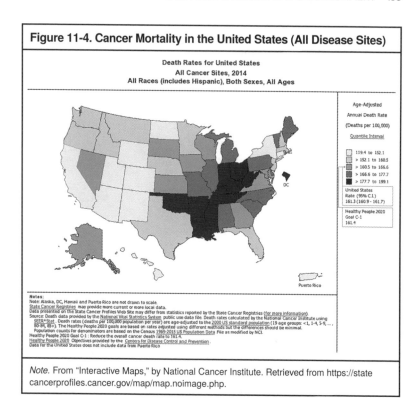

Figure 11-4. Cancer Mortality in the United States (All Disease Sites)

Note. From "Interactive Maps," by National Cancer Institute. Retrieved from https://state cancerprofiles.cancer.gov/map/map.noimage.php.

sure linked to melanoma is a worldwide issue. Global malignant melanoma incidence is approximately 130,000 cases annually. An estimated 66,000 people will die each year from all forms of skin cancer. Food quality, particularly the presence of arsenic in food and drinking water, is a potential contributor to skin, bladder, and lung cancer globally. Table 11-1 lists cancers and their associated environmental contributors on a global scale.

Environmental Considerations in Your Home

The home environment can expose you to chemicals that can affect your health. In fact, some chemicals found in your home are known to increase your risk for cancer. What follows are some

Table 11-1. Evidence-Based Environmental Contributors to Cancer Occurrence	
Cancer Type	**Known Environmental Contributor**
Bladder cancer	Arsenic exposure in drinking water
Leukemia	Exposure to benzene, ethylene oxide, and ionizing radiation
Lung cancer	Exposure to asbestos, arsenic, and other carcinogens Indoor radon exposure Outdoor air pollution Secondhand smoke Solid fuels used for cooking and heating
Skins cancers (including melanoma and basal and squamous cell carcinomas)	Ultraviolet radiation
Stomach cancer	*Helicobacter pylori* transmitted through contaminated food and water
Note. Based on information from World Health Organization, 2011b.	

common sources of potential cancer-causing agents found in the home.

The Water You Drink

Most Americans consume water from public water sources that have standards for safety to protect against contamination. However, approximately 15% of Americans rely on private well water, which has a higher risk for contamination by carcinogens. The most harmful carcinogen found in water is arsenic, which is a semi-metallic element present in rocks and soil, as well as water that comes into contact with these things. Arsenic is odorless and tasteless, and many symptoms of exposure remain unnoticed for a long time. Exposure to arsenic in drinking water is more common in regions where the bedrock contains unusually high levels of arsenic. In the United States, these regions include areas in New Hampshire, Maine, Michigan, and other areas in the Southwest and Rocky Mountains. Many studies have linked arsenic to cancers of the liver, lung, bladder, and kidney. The key to avoiding the long-term effects of arsenic is avoiding exposure.

You can use several methods to reduce your arsenic exposure risk:

- Test private well water for arsenic every year. State governments can provide a list of certified water testing laboratories. Your local health department may also provide private well testing. The U.S. Environmental Protection Agency (EPA) provides an online directory by state of resources for well water safety (see www.epa.gov). Additionally, you can contact state laboratories that are certified to test drinking water for arsenic.
- Avoid boiling or bleaching (using chlorine disinfection) arsenic-containing water supplies. These methods are not strong enough to remove arsenic and may make the levels worse.
- Consider methods to remove arsenic from your home's water supply such as reverse osmosis, ultrafiltration, distillation, or ion exchange. Some of these methods require a filtration system to be installed in your home and can provide clean water for an entire house or a single tap.

FACT OR FICTION: Fluoride in drinking water can lead to cancer.

Fiction. Many studies have been done and have found no strong proof that fluoride in drinking water increases the risk of cancer. Some studies suggested a connection between osteosarcoma (a type of bone cancer) and fluoride use; however, there was not enough evidence to prove a link.

The Air You Breathe

Radon

It has been widely discussed in this book that smoking is the leading cause of lung cancer. However, radon exposure causes the most lung cancer among nonsmokers, according to EPA. Overall, radon is the second leading cause of lung cancer in the United States. Radon is responsible for approximately 21,000 lung cancer deaths every year, and roughly 2,900 of those deaths occur among people who have never smoked. Radon is a colorless, odorless radioactive gas, which makes it difficult to detect through our senses alone. Radon forms as a result of the decay or breakdown of natural radioactive elements in our environment. For example, uranium, which is found in certain soil and rocks, will eventually decay to become radon and other elements. Radon gas in the soil and rocks can move into the air and into ground and surface water.

Chapter 9 discusses the sources and risks of radon in further detail. Because it can enter buildings through the foundation, basements or crawl spaces usually have the highest concentration. Radon exposure can also occur from some building materials. Almost any building material made from natural substances, including concrete and drywall, may give off some amount radon. In most cases these levels are very low, but in a few instances these materials may contribute significantly to radon exposure.

As discussed in Chapter 9, you can perform a do-it-yourself radon detection test. EPA recommends testing below the third floor in all homes. If the results show high levels, radon reduction systems can be installed that can lower radon levels by up to 99%. In general, these systems cost approximately $2,000 to install.

FACT OR FICTION: **Granite countertops increase the risk for radon-induced cancer.**

Fiction. Some granite countertops may expose people to different levels of radon. Most health and radiation experts agree that although a small portion of granite countertops might give off increased levels of radon, most countertops give off extremely low levels. According to EPA, it's very unlikely that a granite countertop in a home would increase the radon level above normal.

Asbestos

Asbestos is a type of mineral that occurs in the environment as bundles of fibers, which are separated into thin, durable threads. These fibers are resistant to heat, fire, and chemicals, and they cannot conduct electricity. Because of these unique properties, asbestos was widely used in construction of homes and buildings in the 20th century. It had numerous applications, such as strengthening cement and plastic, insulation, roofing, fireproofing, and sound absorption.

Studies have shown that asbestos exposure is closely linked with the development of mesothelioma, a form of cancer that most often affects the **pleura** (the thin lining of the organs in the chest) and the **peritoneum** (the thin lining of the organs in the abdomen). In addition, studies have shown that inhaling asbestos is linked to an increased risk of lung cancer. Studies have also found a link between asbestos exposure and increased risk of ovarian, pharyngeal, stomach, laryngeal, and colorectal cancers.

Inhaling or ingesting large amounts of asbestos fibers over a long period of time cause asbestos-related cancers. People who develop asbestos-related diseases do not show symptoms until 10–40 years after the first exposure. For pleural mesothelioma and asbestos-related cancers found in the lung and larynx, symptoms include difficulty breathing, shortness of breath, coughing, and chest pain. Abdominal swelling, pain, indigestion, and changes in bowel habits can occur in peritoneal mesothelioma or asbestos-related cancers of the gastrointestinal tract and ovaries.

People can come in contact with asbestos in their homes by inhaling asbestos particles that become lodged in the clothing of family members who work in places with high levels of asbestos. In addition, living in homes or buildings that contain asbestos may risk exposure. When building materials that contain asbestos—insulation, ceiling, or floor tiles—decompose over time or are disturbed by remodeling or drilling, asbestos fibers can be released into the air.

The U.S. Consumer Product Safety Commission banned the use of asbestos in wallboard patching compounds and gas fireplaces in the late 1970s. It was found that asbestos fibers in these products could be released into the environment during use. In addition, EPA banned all new uses of asbestos in 1989.

Despite the prevalence of asbestos, you can reduce your risk for exposure in your home. If you live in a house built before 1975, check with an asbestos expert, who is specially trained to handle asbestos, and assess if your home has any asbestos material in it. This might include testing the air for asbestos levels. If asbestos needs to be removed from your home, hire qualified contractors to avoid contamination or cause further exposure to family members. If you work in an environment that has potential exposure to asbestos, maintain proper protective gear while working.

If you have been exposed to asbestos, try to determine the level of exposure. Contact with low amounts for short periods of time may carry low risk of developing cancer. High levels of asbestos exposure or exposure for long periods of time may present the greatest danger to health. Studies have shown an increase in mesothelioma and lung cancer in smokers exposed to asbestos, so if you are a smoker, you should quit. Talk to your healthcare provider to see if you should have screening tests such as an x-ray or computed tomography (commonly known as CT) scan to detect cancer. It is important to know the possible symptoms of mesothelioma and lung cancer, including shortness of breath, cough, coughing up blood, chest pain, difficulty swallowing, and weight loss.

Secondhand Smoke

Chapter 6 thoroughly addresses how smoking affects health. However, even if you are not a smoker, you may be at risk if you live with someone who does smoke. Secondhand smoke is any smoke produced by burning a tobacco product. It can also be referred to as *environmental smoke, involuntary smoke,* and *passive smoke.* Of the many harmful substances identified in secondhand smoke, at least 69 are carcinogens. At least 3,000 lung cancer deaths each year in the United States are a direct result of secondhand smoke. The U.S. Surgeon General has noted that people living with a smoker have a 20%–30% higher chance of developing lung cancer. Some research also shows evidence that secondhand smoke may increase the risk of other cancers, such as breast or head and neck cancers in adults, or leukemia, lymphoma, and brain tumors in children.

FACT OR FICTION: Keeping a green lawn free of bugs and other pests increases the risk for cancer.

Fiction. The scientific community has done many studies on fertilizers, pesticides, and other chemicals used to maintain a green and pest-free yard. Studies have shown that typical exposure to these chemicals poses little cancer risk (see Table 11-2).

Table 11-2. Cancer Risks Associated With Household Products	
Product	**Can It Cause Cancer?**
Alcoholic beverages	Yes. Several studies have shown those who regularly consume alcoholic beverages are more likely to develop cancer than those who don't.
Talc powder	Possibly. Based on limited evidence from human studies of a link to ovarian cancer, the International Agency for Research on Cancer classifies the perineal (genital) use of talc-based body powder as "possibly carcinogenic to humans." This substance has garnered much attention recently because lawsuits have been brought against a major manufacturer for talc's possible link to ovarian cancer. It is important to note that each case of ovarian cancer with a possible link to talc needs to be evaluated individually.
Volatile organic compounds (VOCs) (paints, cleaning products, air fresheners)	Possibly. Chemicals found in many VOCs are labeled as carcinogenic. One study has linked a higher rate of breast cancer risk in those who used cleaning supplies and air fresheners containing VOCs than in those who did not. Additional research is needed to further validate a correlation between certain agents and cancers.

(Continued on next page)

Table 11-2. Cancer Risks Associated With Household Products (Continued)	
Product	**Can It Cause Cancer?**
Unused birth control pills or hormone replacement pills	Possibly. Improper disposal of these medications, such as flushing down the toilet or the sink, can release hormones into the surrounding water supply. This can bring potential danger to those who use a public water supply.
Plastic products	Some products, possibly. Research strongly suggests that at certain exposure levels, some of the chemicals in plastic products, such as bisphenol A (BPA), may cause cancer in people.
Cosmetics	Not likely. Although some cosmetic products do contain ingredients (parabens, phthalates) that are thought to be linked to the development of cancer, not enough long-term studies exist to link the application of these products and cancer risk.
Hair dyes	Not likely. At this time, there is not enough research on the long-term effects of hair dyes to prove that there is an increased risk for cancer. However, there is a need for further research.
Antiperspirants	Not likely. No long-term studies have linked cancer and antiperspirant use, and little scientific evidence exists to support the claim. However, more research is needed to better understand this risk.

Note. Based on information from American Cancer Society, 2014, 2016b; Breastcancer.org, n.d.-a, n.d.-b; Doheny, 2008; National Cancer Institute, 2013, 2016a; Zota et al., 2010.

Wood-Burning Fireplaces and Stoves

Many studies have examined the safety of fireplaces and their association with cancer. In most modern homes across the United States, fireplaces now have proper ventilation systems, which remove harmful pollution from the home. However, pollution from use of indoor stoves or fireplaces is a significant source of ambient polycyclic aromatic hydrocarbons (PAHs), which are chemicals produced from burning materials such as wood or coal. Indoor stoves and fireplaces can also emit other cancer-causing substances, such as benzene, formaldehyde, and acrolein.

A 2014 study in *Environmental Health* suggested that emission of PAHs may be linked to certain cancers, such as breast cancer. The burning of synthetic logs in fireplaces posed the most risk. Women who burned synthetic logs were 45% more likely to have breast cancer than those who did not.

Some studies have also suggested that air pollutants from soot resulting from burning wood can lead to cancer. Additionally, those who work as chimney sweeps have a higher rate of scrotal, lung, esophageal, and bladder cancers. Some of these risks can also apply to people who have wood-burning fireplaces and stoves in their homes.

You can minimize your cancer-related risk associated with fireplaces and wood-burning stoves by choosing an EPA-certified appliance. As of May 15, 2015, wood and pellet stoves, fire inserts, outdoor wood boilers, and forced-air furnaces must meet EPA regulatory emission requirements.

FACT OR FICTION: Are "green" products better or safer?

Not necessarily. Ingredients found in common household cleaning products can cause eye irritation, respiratory problems, endocrine problems, and cancer. Therefore, companies have marketed "green" products claiming to be natural, nontoxic, and biodegradable as the better option. Being "green" does not mean those cleaners do not pose any health or environmental risks. The cleaning product market is unregulated. You should read all labels and research the ingredients in the cleaners you use.

Separating evidence-based risk (such as alcohol) from fiction (such as antiperspirants) related to the products you use can support healthy and safe use of everyday products. Scientific evidence shows the relationship between substances and products in our homes with the occurrence of cancer. However, we can control our exposure to many common carcinogens. Testing water for arsenic levels or air for radon and asbestos can increase your awareness and the ability to reduce exposure if these chemicals are present. Additionally, keeping your home and car free from secondhand smoke can greatly reduce cancer risk.

Environmental Considerations in the Workplace

A *workplace environment* is defined as the surrounding conditions in which an employee operates. These conditions can expose people to a variety of hazards, some of which may increase the risk for cancer. The Occupational Safety and Health Administration (OSHA) identifies a number of health and safety hazard categories, and four can be linked to cancer risk:

- Chemical and dust hazards may expose a worker to various states of chemicals, including solid, liquid, or gas. Although some may be safer than others, chemicals create sensitivities or can cause damage to the cells after exposure.
- Biologic hazards are present while working with people, animals, or infectious agents.
- Physical hazards such as heat, radiation, and noise can cause harm without direct contact to the employee.
- Work organization hazards include the high-stress demands of a job, including shift work hours and workload.

Exposure to all types of hazards may happen through inhalation, ingestion, absorption, or injection. Some occupations have an increased cancer risk based on the level and length of exposure. A list of evidence-based relationships between workplace exposures, professions, and cancer is listed in Table 11-3.

Based on research, the most common danger related to cancer in the workplace is breathing in chemicals and dust, followed by absorption through the skin. The rate of lung and blood cancers among the jobs listed is higher, possibly because of inhalation as the main route of exposure.

Duration of exposure also factors into cancer risk. Exposure may be acute or chronic. *Acute exposure* is defined as hav-

Table 11-3. Cancer Exposures Based on Occupation		
Type of Cancer	**Occupation**	**Hazard Category**
Bladder	Firefighters, roofers, cosmetologists	Chemical and dust
Breast	Plant workers, nurses, night shift workers, astronauts, flight crews	Chemical and dust, physical, workplace organization
Cholangiocarcinoma (gallbladder cancer)	Printers	Chemical and dust
Colorectal	Farmers/agricultural workers, night shift workers, astronauts, plant workers	Chemical and dust, physical, workplace organization
Digestive tract	Roofers, plant workers	Chemical and dust
Esophagus	Plant workers, miners	Chemical and dust
Kidney	Firefighters, roofers, plant workers	Chemical and dust, physical
Leukemia	Farmers/agricultural workers, healthcare workers, astronauts	Chemical and dust, physical
Liver	Plant workers	Chemical and dust
Lung	Farmers/agricultural workers, firefighters, roofers, cosmetologists, sheet metal workers, metal workers, plastics/machine operators, electrical and electronic equipment assemblers, radiologic technicians, health technologists and technicians, engineering and chemical technicians, administrative support, equipment manufacturing workers, radio/television communication workers, astronauts, miners, plant workers	Chemical and dust, physical, workplace organization
Non-Hodgkin lymphoma	Farmers/agricultural workers, cosmetologists	Chemical and dust

(Continued on next page)

Table 11-3. Cancer Exposures Based on Occupation *(Continued)*		
Type of Cancer	Occupation	Hazard Category
Prostate	Farmers/agricultural workers, firefighters, night shift workers	Chemical and dust, physical, workplace organization
Skin	Nurses, firefighters, roofers, flight crews	Chemical and dust, physical
Thyroid	Cosmetologists, astronauts	Chemical and dust, physical

ing a large, single dose in a short time period. *Chronic exposure* is defined as having many doses over a long period of time. Several organizations, including OSHA and the American Conference of Governmental Industrial Hygienists, have established exposure limits for hazards. These limits are based on an eight-hour work shift in which the highest level of exposure for the average employee will not cause harm. The employee and the work environment may be monitored through industrial practices to determine exposure, and results may show the need for controls.

Night Shift Work: A Case Study

Recent studies have shown a link between female night shift workers and breast cancer incidence. Contact with bright light at night causes decreased melatonin and impacts the production of estrogen. The suppression of estrogen production can lead to an increased risk of breast cancer. Data have shown that women who frequently work 12-hour rotating shifts, alternating from day to night, have a higher rate of breast cancer than women who work shorter, more consistent shifts. This is a significant number of people, as approximately 15% of the U.S. workforce works night shift hours. Although there appears to be some association with cancer from the effects of disruptions in melatonin production, these other possible consequences of night shift work should be studied further:

- Chronic disruption of the timing of sleep (phase shift sleep disruption)
- Changes in metabolism
- Desynchronization between the central and peripheral nervous systems
- Decreased vitamin D production

Reducing Risk of Exposure: The Hierarchy of Controls

The *hierarchy of controls* in the workplace is a set of methods to reduce exposure to hazardous materials (see Figure 11-5). These options are used to eliminate or minimize the exposure to hazards:

- *Engineering controls* remove the hazard at the source before the worker can become exposed. For example, a fume hood in a

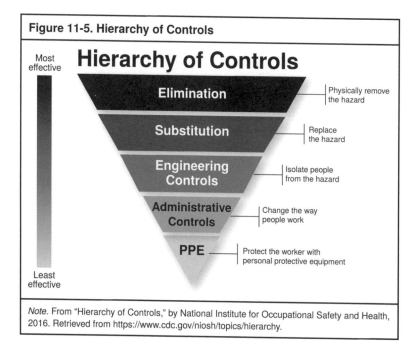

Figure 11-5. Hierarchy of Controls

Hierarchy of Controls

Most effective

Elimination	Physically remove the hazard
Substitution	Replace the hazard
Engineering Controls	Isolate people from the hazard
Administrative Controls	Change the way people work
PPE	Protect the worker with personal protective equipment

Least effective

Note. From "Hierarchy of Controls," by National Institute for Occupational Safety and Health, 2016. Retrieved from https://www.cdc.gov/niosh/topics/hierarchy.

laboratory ventilates chemical vapors away from an employee's breathing zone to reduce exposure.

- *Administrative controls* are changes in work procedures, such as written safety policies, rules, supervision, schedules, and training.
- *Personal protective equipment* can be worn to reduce exposure to workplace hazards. Examples include respirators, gloves, face shields, and coveralls.

Together, these controls reduce the risk of cancer and illness. While it is important to reduce hazards, an effective safety program will continue to evaluate the safety culture and promote a safe workplace. OSHA and other regulatory agencies, along with state and local health departments, play a key role in guiding employers to maintain a safe and healthy workplace. Effective workplaces support a safety culture that protects employees through the approval, endorsement, and enforcement of health regulations.

Controlling Hazards: Personal Accountability

Education on controlling hazards is an important part of a successful safety program. Employees exposed to chemicals or dust that are not controlled with ventilation need to understand their exposures. Additionally, coworkers and managers need to be held accountable for safety practices.

Sometimes, repetitive activities can begin to seem commonplace and attention to safety guidelines can be forgotten. Ensuring that exposures are limited through consistent and standardized hazard controls, particularly the use of personal protective equipment, is critical to reducing exposure risk.

For example, in a dentist's office, a dental hygienist may not always wear a lead apron or place one on the patient when performing x-rays. If another hygienist or the dentist does not require this practice, unnecessary radiation exposures will occur to patients and employees. It can be a challenge to enforce the consistent use of personal protective equipment. Time, reduced perception of risk, or lack of education about the reason for the safety behaviors can contribute to noncompliance and risk for exposures that may cause cancer. Workplace leaders should set and model the expectation for workplace safety. However, every employee should also understand the risks for exposure and how to reduce them.

Exposure, duration, and lack of controls collectively contribute to the increased risk of cancer from workplace hazards but can be reduced through an effective safety program. Identifying hazards and using evidence-based standards are critical to reducing risk in the workplace. In addition, everyone must be held accountable and take responsibility to maintain a safe work environment. If you are aware of risky conditions or behaviors, notify your supervisor. If the condition does not improve, you have the right to share your concern with someone higher up in the organization until safe conditions are reestablished (see Figure 11-6).

Figure 11-6. Key Questions to Ask Employers/Employees About Organizational Health

• Who is responsible for safety at your company?
• Who is responsible for assessing risk at your company?
• Were safety expectations set when you were first hired?
• Is safety a part of your evaluation process?

Environmental Considerations in Our Communities

The Air You Breathe

The International Agency for Research on Cancer has identified outdoor air pollution as a carcinogen. Much of the research studying outdoor air pollution has shown that exposure can lead to lung and bladder cancers, among others. Outdoor air pollution includes any **particulate matter**, classified as chemical, mechanical, or a combination of both.

Fossil fuel power plants, steel mills, and diesel- or gasoline-powered motor vehicles are common sources of chemical particulate matter. Common examples of mechanical particulate matter are dust particles and construction and demolition debris. Mining operations and agriculture operations contribute mechanical particulate matter to air pollution. The next section will discuss some of the common sources of air pollution and the impact they may have on cancer risk.

Traffic Exhaust

A large amount of research points to a connection between cancer and exposure to traffic exhaust. These fumes may contain known carcinogens, such as soot, heavy metals, sulfur dioxide, nitrogen oxide, and other volatile compounds. A 2015 *Environmental Health Perspectives* study showed high levels of nitrogen oxide in traffic exhaust that was linked to an increased occurrence of lung cancer in people who were exposed to the fumes more often. Other studies also show relationships between lung and other cancers and how close a location is to traffic exhaust. Although the exact cause of the relationship between exhaust fumes and cancer may be hard to identify, the World Health Organization recommends taking measures to limit exposure to traffic exhaust fuels. If you live in a high-traffic area with exposure to exhaust air pollution, you may consider these measures:

- Staying indoors when possible, especially during times of high air pollution levels
- Leaving car windows up during commutes on busy roads
- Minimizing children's time outdoors when air pollution levels are highest

September 11, 2001, Brings a Lifetime of Concern for Cancer Risk: A Case Study

No one can forget the amazing bravery shown by the first responders who risked their lives to save others in the September 11 attacks on the World Trade Center. However, the men and women who escaped the devastation with their lives now face a lifetime of risks for cancer related to this horrific day in history. The September 11 attacks represent one of the greatest environmental hazard exposures in American history. Particle dust, soot, exhaust from burning jet fuel, and large amounts of asbestos were released into the environment. The Mesothelioma Center has detailed the impact that this asbestos exposure may have on those involved; see www.asbestos.com/world-trade-center for further information.

Fossil Fuel Power Plants

Fossil fuel power plants burn coal, oil, or gas to create steam in a combustion chamber. The chemicals released during combustion can potentially cause cancer. Benzene, a known carcinogen, is one of the largest-volume petrochemical solvents used in the fossil fuel industry. A vast amount of research links benzene exposure to development of leukemia, multiple myeloma, and non-Hodgkin lymphoma.

Electromagnetic Fields

Electric and magnetic fields are areas of energy invisible to the human eye. An electric field is produced by voltage, and a magnetic field is a result of currents flowing through wires or electronic devices. Together, they are known as *electromagnetic fields* (EMFs). EMF types include high-frequency EMFs (ionizing radiation), which include x-rays and gamma rays, and low to moderate EMFs (nonionizing radiation), which include magnetic fields from electric power lines and appliances, radio waves, microwaves, and infrared radiation.

High-frequency EMFs pose the greatest risk for the development of cancer because they are part of the electromagnetic spectrum that can directly damage cells and DNA. Overall, current research states that low to moderate EMF exposure poses little risk of cancer. Research is ongoing as each of these technologies advance.

FACT OR FICTION: Using electronics such as microwaves, cell phones, cordless phones, and Wi-Fi devices can cause cancer.

Unknown. In 2002, the International Agency for Research on Cancer, a component of the World Health Organization, appointed an expert Working Group to review all available evidence on static and extremely low-frequency EMFs. The Working Group classified extremely low-frequency EMFs as "possibly carcinogenic to humans" based on limited examples from studies about childhood leukemia. The group determined that static electric and magnetic fields and extremely low-frequency electric fields were "not classifiable as to their carcinogenicity to humans." The American Cancer Society suggests that there could be some cancer risk associated with radiofrequency energy, but the evidence is not yet strong enough, and more investigation is necessary.

Soil Pollution

Although we often take for granted the importance of what's below our feet, soil can be an important aspect of our overall health and well-being. Just like in many other elements of nature, soil pollution occurs when man-made substances contaminate it. Soil pollution has several common sources:

- Industrial activities—Many industries extract minerals from the earth, such as iron or coal, and the by-products of this process contaminate the soil.
- Agricultural activities—The use of pesticides and fertilizers has been on the rise. These chemicals cannot be broken down and eventually seep into the soil, decreasing the fertility of the soil. Plants absorb these harmful chemicals, resulting in potentially harmful effects from consumption of the foods harvested from this soil.
- Waste disposal—The way we dispose of waste is a huge concern, especially regarding soil pollution. Whether it is chemical or human waste, our sewer systems can be a vehicle to soil pollution. The carcinogen benzene, a common waste product, has been linked to leukemia. Another set of pollutants, polychlo-

rinated biphenyls (commonly known as PCBs), may cause liver cancer.

Water Pollution

Access to clean water is at the very foundation of human survival. The processes used to purify water of bacteria and other harmful agents determine whether a water supply is safe for drinking and bathing. EPA requires all municipal water utilities to disinfect raw water supplies. Before this policy began, outbreaks of serious diseases such as typhoid fever, cholera, and dysentery were common causes of death in the United States. Although today we do not worry much about contracting a disease from drinking municipal water, some concern exists about disinfectant by-products (DBPs)—unwanted substances formed when disinfectants, such as chlorine, react with organic matter in drinking water. Beginning in the 1970s, scientists noticed there were low levels of DBPs in drinking water. This discovery led to regulation of the amount of DBPs in the water supply and further investigation of the long-term effects of DBP exposure. Several studies examined the relationship between gastrointestinal and urinary cancers and DBP exposure. Many of these studies concluded that the risk of exposure to dangerous pathogens in untreated water is far more dangerous than the possible low cancer risk that DBP consumption poses.

Superfund Sites

Hazardous waste can be in the form of a liquid, a solid, or sludge. It is often generated from manufacturing plants, repair shops, hospitals, laboratories, construction sites, and our homes. Hazardous waste, if not disposed of properly, may poison water sources and cause ground contamination that can lead to breast cancer and leukemia. EPA has established requirements that companies and individuals must abide by to manage how hazardous waste is handled, treated, and ultimately disposed of. In the past, hazardous waste was not controlled and was often dumped illegally, especially in low-income communities. In 1980, the Comprehensive Environmental Response, Compensation, and Liability Act (CERCLA or Superfund) became law and gave EPA control over cleaning up these sites and reclaiming the land for reuse and development. If you witness illegal dumping, contact the authorities and report it. Even everyday citizens can help keep the environment safe from toxins that pollute our water, soil, and air.

Summary

Many factors in our homes, communities, and workplaces can potentially affect our cancer risk. With knowledge of the potential harms that can be found in our outside environment, we can significantly decrease or even eliminate exposure to carcinogens. With knowledge of what pollutants are present in our air, water, and soil, we can make more informed decisions about where we choose to live, grow our foods, and spend our time enjoying the outdoors. The challenge in our communities is that many of the potential hazards cannot be seen by the naked eye. To protect ourselves and our families from increased cancer risks, we must continually educate ourselves on potential threats.

Whether at home, at work, or in the community, we are constantly interacting within these environments that contain many substances that can contribute to the development of cancer. Although some exposures are outside of our control, there are ways we can safely engage in the environments around us. Knowing what we can control, such as sun and tobacco exposure, and limiting these factors can reduce cancer risk. Taking precautions to test our homes for radon in the air and arsenic in the water also reduces the chances of cancer. Workers should be familiar with job environments and safety standards regarding hazardous materials, particularly in healthcare and industrial settings. When necessary, they should use personal protective equipment thoughtfully and in compliance with national guidelines. Finally, everyone should familiarize themselves with community-based risks, including water sources, soil, and potential air pollutants. Although we ultimately cannot control every exposure, we can eliminate some risks and reduce others. Doing so can ensure we continue to live happy, healthy, and thriving lives while engaging with the many environments around us.

Recommended Reading

Asbestos.com. (2016). Asbestos, 9/11 air toxins related to cancer. Retrieved from https://www.asbestos.com/world-trade-center

National Cancer Institute. (2015). Environmental carcinogens and cancer risk. Retrieved from https://www.cancer.gov/about-cancer/causes -prevention/risk/substances/carcinogens

Simon, S. (2013). World Health Organization: Outdoor air pollution causes cancer. Retrieved from https://www.cancer.org/latest-news/world-health -organization-outdoor-air-pollution-causes-cancer.html

World Health Organization. (2016). Air pollution levels rising in many of the world's poorest cities. Retrieved from http://www.who.int/mediacentre /news/releases/2016/air-pollution-rising/en

Glossary

particulate matter—Material suspended in the air in the form of minute solid particles or liquid droplets, especially when considered as an atmospheric pollutant.

peritoneum [payr-ih-toh-nee-um]—The tissue that lines the abdominal wall and covers most of the organs in the abdomen.

pleura [ploor-uh]—A thin layer of tissue that covers the lungs and lines the interior wall of the chest cavity. It protects and cushions the lungs. This tissue secretes a small amount of fluid that acts as a lubricant, allowing the lungs to move smoothly in the chest cavity while breathing.

The authors gratefully acknowledge the contributions of Amy Sisson, Research Librarian, for her skillful gathering and organization of references, and Matthew Berkheiser, Executive Director of Environmental Health and Safety; Lynette Leadon, Director of Environmental Health and Safety; Elena McLaughlin, Principal Safety Specialist; and Sandra Jimenez, Radiation Safety Officer, all in the Department of Environmental Health and Safety at The University of Texas MD Anderson Cancer Center, for their contributions to this chapter.

Appendices

Appendix A. Resources

General
Dictionary.com: www.dictionary.com
The Free Dictionary, medical: http://medical-dictionary.thefreedictionary.com
MedicineNet.com: www.medicinenet.com/script/main/hp.asp

Cancer
American Cancer Society: www.cancer.org
American Institute for Cancer Research: www.aicr.org
Livestrong Foundation: www.livestrong.org
National Cancer Institute: www.cancer.gov
National Cancer Institute Dictionaries: www.cancer.gov/publications/dictionaries
Susan G. Komen: ww5.komen.org

Environment
Centers for Disease Control and Prevention's *Cancer Prevention During Early Life*
    video: www.youtube.com/watch?v=pt_chxEi42Y
Environmental Protection Agency: www.epa.gov

Food and Nutrition
The Center for Mindful Eating: www.thecenterformindfuleating.org
My Food My Health: http://myfoodmyhealth.com (Low-cost meal planning website
    that provides recipes appropriate for a variety of dietary restrictions and can cre-
    ate a shopping list)
Rebecca Katz: www.rebeccakatz.com (Katz translates nutritional science into flavor-
    ful, everyday recipes to improve health; includes recipes, videos, and more)

Genetics
GeneReviews: www.ncbi.nlm.nih.gov/books/NBK1116 (Searchable database with
    detailed information about genetic syndromes)

National Cancer Institute: The genetics of cancer: www.cancer.gov/cancertopics/
genetics (Patient information on genetics and cancer)
National Human Genome Research Institute: www.genome.gov
• Policy, legal, and ethical issues in genetics: www.genome.gov/issues
• Talking Glossary of Genetic Terms: www.genome.gov/glossary
National Library of Medicine Genetics Home Reference: https://ghr.nlm.nih.gov
(Consumer information about many genetic conditions)
National Society of Genetic Counselors: www.nsgc.org (Searchable database to
find a credentialed genetics professional by zip code)

Heart and Lung Health
American Heart Association: www.heart.org
American Liver Foundation: www.liverfoundation.org
American Lung Association: www.lung.org
National Institute on Alcohol Abuse and Alcoholism: www.niaaa.nih.gov
Smokefree.gov: https://smokefree.gov (A free national tobacco cessation resource)
U.S. Surgeon General: www.surgeongeneral.gov

Hereditary Cancer Syndromes
Bright Pink: www.brightpink.org (Source of online and other support services for
young women affected by a diagnosis of breast or ovarian cancer)
FORCE (Facing Our Risk of Cancer Empowered): www.facingourrisk.org/index.php
(Source of online and local support for women with hereditary breast and ovarian
cancer syndromes)
Hereditary Colon Cancer Takes Guts: www.hcctakesguts.org (Information and
online support for families with a variety of types of hereditary colon cancer syndromes)
My Family Health Portrait®: Patient and caregiver resources: https://familyhistory
.hhs.gov/FHH/html/index.html (A tool for assessing risk through family history)
National Comprehensive Cancer Network: www.nccn.org/patients/default.aspx (Provides searchable guidelines for testing and management for people with hereditary risk for developing cancer)
Sharsheret: http://sharsheret.org (Information and support for people of Jewish
ancestry affected by hereditary cancer syndromes)

Vaccinations
Healthcare.gov vaccination insurance coverage assistance: www.healthcare.gov
Vaccines for Children program: www.cdc.gov/vaccines/programs/vfc/index.html

Appendix B. Cancer Screening Tools

Standard Body Map

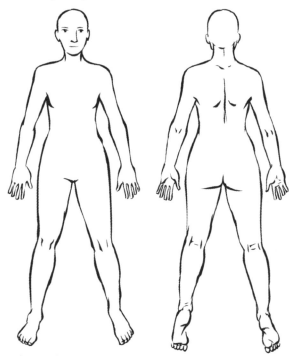

You can use the standard body map to pinpoint and keep track of freckles, moles, or other skin changes as you do your skin assessments. Use a comb or brush to check your scalp, and use a mirror or a partner to view all areas of your body. Document what you see via the ABCDE method; see Chapters 2 and 3 for additional information. Remember to take your body map to your primary care provider or dermatology appointments.

Note. From "Body Maps," by The Skin Cancer Foundation, 2016. Retrieved from http://www .skincancer.org/Media/Default/File/File/scf-body-map-2016.pdf. Copyright 2016 by The Skin Cancer Foundation. Reprinted with permission.

Family Cancer Screening Table

Keeping track of all family members' cancer screenings can be daunting. Use the table to identify family members, their respective screening tests, dates of completion, and dates when future tests are needed per healthcare professional discussions and recommendations.

Cancer	Type of Screening Test	Date of Last Completed Test	Date Next Test Needed
Name:			
Skin			
Breast			
Prostate			
Lung			
Colorectal			
Cervical			
Name:			
Skin			
Breast			
Prostate			
Lung			
Colorectal			
Cervical			
Name:			
Skin			
Breast			
Prostate			
Lung			
Colorectal			
Cervical			
Name:			
Skin			
Breast			
Prostate			
Lung			
Colorectal			
Cervical			

Screening Tools by Cancer

Type of Cancer	Screening Tool
Adrenal cancer	No approved tests currently
Anal cancer	No approved tests currently Men older than age 50 should have an annual rectal examination.
Bladder cancer	No approved tests currently Hematuria test to identify blood in urine is sometimes used.
Brain cancer	No approved tests currently
Breast cancer	Breast self-examination Breast ultrasound Clinical breast examination Magnetic resonance imaging (MRI) Mammography Tomosynthesis (digital mammography)
Cervical cancer	Papanicolaou (Pap) test
Colon cancer	Camera pill Colonoscopy Double-contrast barium enema (DCBE) Fecal immunochemical test (FIT or iFOBT) Flexible sigmoidoscopy High-sensitivity fecal occult blood test (FOBT) Stool DNA Virtual colonoscopy
Endometrial cancer	No approved tests currently
Esophageal cancer	No approved tests currently
Gastrointestinal stromal tumor (GIST)	No approved tests currently
Kidney cancer	No approved tests currently
Leukemia	No approved tests currently
Lung cancer	Low-dose computed tomography (LDCT) scan
Lymphoma	No approved tests currently
Multiple myeloma (cancer of blood plasma cells)	No approved tests currently
Osteosarcoma (bone cancer)	No approved tests currently

Type of Cancer	Screening Tool
Ovarian cancer	No approved tests currently Women at risk have been tested with cancer antigen 125 (CA-125) tumor marker and transvaginal ultrasound.
Pancreatic cancer	No approved tests currently
Prostate cancer	Prostate-specific antigen test (PSA) Digital rectal examination (DRE) Watchful waiting
Retinoblastoma (cancer of retina)	Red reflex examination
Skin cancer	Skin check
Testicular cancer	No approved tests currently
Thyroid cancer	No approved tests currently

Appendix C. References

Chapter 1. Overview of Cancer

Amuta, A.O., & Barry, A.E. (2015). Influence of family history of cancer on engagement in protective health behaviors. *American Journal of Health Education, 46,* 157–164. doi:10.1080/19325037.2015.1023478

Anisimov, V.N. (2007). Biology of aging and cancer. *Cancer Control, 14,* 23–31.

Gustafson, S.L., Raymond, V.M., Marvin, M.L., Else, T., Koeppe, E., Stoffel, E.M., & Everett, J.N. (2015). Outcomes of genetic evaluation for hereditary cancer syndromes in unaffected individuals. *Familial Cancer, 14,* 167–174. doi:10.1007/s10689-014-9756-x

Henderson, B.E., & Feigelson, H.S. (2000). Hormonal carcinogenesis. *Carcinogenesis, 21,* 427–433.

Nacos, G.A. (n.d.). A message from our founder. Retrieved from http://cedarsdragons.ca/cedarscansupport-ca

Rieger, P.T. (2006). Cancer biology and implications for practice. *Clinical Journal of Oncology Nursing, 10,* 457–460. doi:10.1188/06.CJON.457-460

Siegel, R.L., Miller, K.D., & Jemal, A. (2017). Cancer statistics, 2017. *CA: A Cancer Journal for Clinicians, 67,* 7–30. doi:10.3322/caac.21387

Skloot, R. (2010). *The immortal life of Henrietta Lacks.* New York, NY: Broadway Books.

Chapter 2. Sun Safety

Agency for Healthcare Research and Quality. (2014). Recommendations for adults. In *Guide to clinical preventive services, 2014* (AHRQ Publication No. 14-05158). Retrieved from https://www.ahrq.gov/professionals/clinicians-providers/guidelines-recommendations/guide/section2.html

American Cancer Society. (2017a). *Cancer facts and figures 2017.* Retrieved from https://www.cancer.org/research/cancer-facts-statistics/all-cancer-facts-figures/cancer-facts-figures-2017.html

American Cancer Society. (2017b). Key statistics for melanoma skin cancer. Retrieved from https://www.cancer.org/cancer/melanoma-skin-cancer/about/key-statistics.html

Centers for Disease Control and Prevention. (2015). *Skin cancer prevention progress report 2015.* Retrieved from https://www.cdc.gov/cancer/skin/what_cdc_is_doing/progress_report.htm

DePietro, M. (2016). Photosensitivity. Retrieved from http://www.healthline.com/health/photosensitivity

Downham, T.F. (1998). The shadow rule: A simple method for sun protection. *Southern Medical Journal, 91,* 619–623.

National Cancer Institute. (2012). Layers of the skin. Retrieved from http://www.training.seer.cancer.gov/melanoma/anatomy/layers.html

National Cancer Institute. (2017a). Cancer statistics. Retrieved from https://www.cancer.gov/about-cancer/understanding/statistics

National Cancer Institute. (2017b). Melanoma treatment (PDQ®) [Health professional version]. Retrieved from http://www.cancer.gov/types/skin/hp/melanoma-treatment-pdq

National Cancer Institute. (2017c). Skin cancer screening (PDQ®) [Patient version]. Retrieved from https://www.cancer.gov/types/skin/patient/skin-treatment-pdq

National Cancer Institute. (2017d). Skin cancer treatment (PDQ®) [Health professional version]. Retrieved from https://www.cancer.gov/types/skin/hp/skin-treatment-pdq

Norval, M., & Wulf, H.C. (2009). Does chronic sunscreen use reduce vitamin D production to insufficient levels? British Journal of Dermatology, 161, 732–736. doi:10.1111/j.1365-2133.2009.09332.x

Rao, J., Bissonnette, R., Taylor, C.R., & Van Voorhees, A.S. (2016). Photodynamic therapy for the dermatologist. Retrieved from http://emedicine.medscape.com/article/1121517-overview

Shafie Pour, N., Saeedi, M., Morteza Semnani, K., & Akbari, J. (2015). Sun protection for children: A review. Journal of Pediatrics Review, 3, e155. doi:10.5812/jpr.155

Skin Cancer Foundation. (n.d.-a). Actinic keratosis (AK). Retrieved from http://www.skincancer.org/skin-cancer-information/actinic-keratosis

Skin Cancer Foundation. (n.d.-b). Basal cell carcinoma (BCC). Retrieved from http://www.skincancer.org/skin-cancer-information/basal-cell-carcinoma

Skin Cancer Foundation. (n.d.-c). Squamous cell carcinoma (SCC). Retrieved from http://www.skincancer.org/skin-cancer-information/squamous-cell-carcinoma

Skin Cancer Foundation. (2012). Melanoma soars among young adults. Retrieved from http://www.skincancer.org/publications/sun-and-skin-news/spring-2012-29-1/melanoma-soars

Skin Cancer Foundation. (2017a). Sun safety tips for infants, babies and toddlers. Retrieved from http://www.skincancer.org/prevention/sun-protection/children/sun-safety-tips-for-infants-babies-and-toddlers

Skin Cancer Foundation. (2017b). UVA and UVB. Retrieved from http://www.skincancer.org/prevention/uva-and-uvb

Tripp, M.K., Watson, M., Balk, S.J., & Swetter, S.M. (2016). State of the science on prevention and screening to reduce melanoma incidence and mortality: The time is now. CA: A Cancer Journal for Clinicians, 66, 460–480. doi:10.3322/caac.21352

U.S. Department of Health and Human Services. (2015). The Surgeon General's call to action to prevent skin cancer. Retrieved from https://www.cdc.gov/cancer/skin/call_to_action/index.htm

U.S. Environmental Protection Agency. (n.d.-a). UV index forecast. Retrieved from https://www.epa.gov/sunsafety/uv-index-1

U.S. Environmental Protection Agency. (n.d.-b). UV index scale. Retrieved from https://www.epa.gov/sunsafety/uv-index-scale-0

U.S. Environmental Protection Agency. (2010). Action steps for sun safety. Retrieved from https://www.epa.gov/sunsafety/action-steps-sun-safety

U.S. Food and Drug Administration. (2017). Sunscreen: How to protect your skin from the sun. Retrieved from https://www.fda.gov/drugs/resourcesforyou/consumers/buyingusingmedicinesafely/understandingover-the-countermedicines/ucm239463.htm

U.S. Preventive Services Task Force. (2016). Final research plan for skin cancer prevention: Behavioral counseling. Retrieved from http://www.uspreventiveservicestaskforce.org/Page/Document/final-research-plan/skin-cancer-counseling2

World Health Organization. (2016). INTERSUN Programme. Retrieved from http://who.int/uv/intersunprogramme/en

Chapter 3. Screening for Cancer

American Academy of Dermatology. (2016). What to expect at a SPOTme® skin cancer screening. Retrieved from https://www.aad.org/public/spot-skin-cancer/programs/screenings/what-to-expect-at-a-screening

American Association for Pediatric Ophthalmology and Strabismus. (2016). Retinoblastoma. Retrieved from https://aapos.org/terms/conditions/93

American Cancer Society. (2015). What are the risk factors for retinoblastoma? Retrieved from http://www.cancer.org/cancer/retinoblastoma/detailedguide/retinoblastoma-risk-factors

American Cancer Society. (2016a). American Cancer Society guidelines for the prevention and early detection of cervical cancer. Retrieved from http://www.cancer.org/cancer/cervicalcancer/moreinformation/cervicalcancerpreventionandearlydetection/cervical-cancer-prevention-and-early-detection-cervical-cancer-screening-guidelines

American Cancer Society. (2016b). American Cancer Society recommendations for prostate cancer early detection. Retrieved from http://www.cancer.org/cancer/prostatecancer/moreinformation/prostatecancerearlydetection/prostate-cancer-early-detection-acs-recommendations

American Cancer Society. (2016c). Can anal cancer be found early? Retrieved from http://www.cancer.org/cancer/analcancer/detailedguide/anal-cancer-detection

American Cancer Society. (2017a). American Cancer Society guidelines for early detection of cancer. Retrieved from http://www.cancer.org/healthy/findcancerearly/cancerscreeningguidelines/american-cancer-society-guidelines-for-the-early-detection-of-cancer

American Cancer Society. (2017b). Key statistics for lung cancer. Retrieved from http://www.cancer.org/cancer/lungcancer-non-smallcell/detailedguide/non-small-cell-lung-cancer-key-statistics

American Cancer Society. (2017c). Key statistics for prostate cancer. Retrieved from http://www.cancer.org/cancer/prostatecancer/detailedguide/prostate-cancer-key-statistics

American Cancer Society. (2017d). What are the key statistics about ovarian cancer? Retrieved from http://www.cancer.org/cancer/ovariancancer/detailedguide/ovarian-cancer-key-statistics

American College of Obstetricians and Gynecologists. (2013). New guidelines for cervical cancer screening. Retrieved from https://www.acog.org/-/media/For-Patients/pfs004.pdf?dmc=1&ts=20160815T1402318142

Breastcancer.org. (2016). Mammography: Benefits, risks, what you need to know. Retrieved from http://www.breastcancer.org/symptoms/testing/types/mammograms/benefits_risks

Cancer Connect. (n.d.). Cancer screening. Retrieved from http://news.cancerconnect.com/testing-center/cancer-screening

Carlson, K. (2017, April 18). Screening for ovarian cancer [Literature review current through June 2017]. Retrieved from http://www.uptodate.com/contents/screening-for-ovarian-cancer

Colon and Rectal Surgery Associates. (n.d.). Abnormal anal pap smear, anal dysplasia and anal cancer. Retrieved from http://www.colorectal.org/services.cfm/sid:7580/Abnormal_Anal_Pap_Smear,_Anal_Dysplasia_and_Anal_Cancer/index.html

National Cancer Institute. (2016a). Bladder and other urothelial cancers screening (PDQ®) [Patient version]. Retrieved from http://www.cancer.gov/types/bladder/patient/bladder-screening-pdq

National Cancer Institute. (2016b). Tests to detect colorectal cancer and polyps. Retrieved from http://www.cancer.gov/types/colorectal/screening-fact-sheet

National Cancer Institute. (2017a). Cancer screening overview (PDQ®) [Patient version]. Retrieved from http://www.cancer.gov/about-cancer/screening/patient-screening-overview-pdq

National Cancer Institute. (2017b). Endometrial cancer screening (PDQ®) [Patient version]. Retrieved from http://www.cancer.gov/types/uterine/patient/endometrial-screening-pdq

National Cancer Institute. (2017c). Lung cancer screening (PDQ®) [Health professional version]. Retrieved from http://www.cancer.gov/types/lung/hp/lung-screening-pdq

National Cancer Institute. (2017d). Prostate-specific antigen (PSA) test. Retrieved from http://www.cancer.gov/types/prostate/psa-fact-sheet

National Comprehensive Cancer Network. (2016). *NCCN Clinical Practice Guidelines in Oncology (NCCN Guidelines®): Genetic/familial high-risk assessment: Breast and ovarian* [v.2.2017]. Retrieved from https://www.nccn.org/professionals/physician_gls/pdf/genetics_screening.pdf

Oeffinger, K.C., Fontham, E.T.H., Etzioni, R., Herzig, A., Michaelson, J.S., Shih, Y.C.T., … Wender, R. (2015). Breast cancer screening for women at average risk: 2015 guideline update from the American Cancer Society. *JAMA, 314,* 1599–1614. doi:10.1001/jama.2015.12783

Saslow, D., Boetes, C., Burke, W., Harms, S., Leach, M.O., Lehman, C.D., … Russell, C.A. (2007). American Cancer Society guidelines for breast screening with MRI as an adjunct to mammography. *CA: A Cancer Journal for Clinicians, 57,* 75–89. doi:10.3322/canjclin.57.2.75

Simon, S. (2017). Colon cancer screening: What are the options? Retrieved from http://www.cancer.org/cancer/news/features/understanding-tests-that-screen-for-colon-cancer.

U.S. Preventive Services Task Force. (2015). Lung cancer: Screening. Retrieved from http://www.uspreventiveservicestaskforce.org/Page/Document/UpdateSummaryFinal/lung-cancer-screening

University of Texas MD Anderson Cancer Center. (n.d.-a). Adrenal tumors. Retrieved from https://www.mdanderson.org/cancer-types/adrenal-tumors.html

University of Texas MD Anderson Cancer Center. (n.d.-b). Anal cancer. Retrieved from https://www.mdanderson.org/cancer-types/anal-cancer.html

Chapter 4. Physical Activity

American Cancer Society. (2016). ACS guidelines on nutrition and physical activity for cancer prevention. Retrieved from https://www.cancer.org/healthy/eat-healthy-get-active/acs-guidelines-nutrition-physical-activity-cancer-prevention.html

AuYoung, M., Linke, S.E., Pagoto, S., Buman, M.P., Craft, L.L., Richardson, C.R., … Gorin, S.S. (2016). Integrating physical activity in primary care practice. *American Journal of Medicine, 129,* 1022–1029. doi:10.1016/j.amjmed.2016.02.008

Centers for Disease Control and Prevention. (2015). Physical activity and health. Retrieved from https://www.cdc.gov/physicalactivity/basics/pa-health/index.htm

Chin, H.G. (2014). Physical activity in women: Current guidelines and strategies for promoting compliance. *Clinical Obstetrics and Gynecology, 57,* 456–464. doi:10 .1097/grf.0000000000000045

Gonçalves, A.K., Florêncio, G.L.D., de Atayde Silva, M.J.M., Cobucci, R.N., Giraldo, P.C., & Cote, N.M. (2014). Effects of physical activity on breast cancer prevention: A systematic review. *Journal of Physical Activity and Health, 11,* 445–454. doi:10 .1123/jpah.2011-0316

Keadle, S.K., Arem, H., Moore, S.C., Sampson, J.N., & Matthews, C.E. (2015). Impact of changes in television viewing time and physical activity on longevity: A prospective cohort study. *International Journal of Behavioral Nutrition and Physical Activity, 12,* 156. doi:10.1186/s12966-015-0315-0

Lemanne, D., Cassileth, B.R., & Gubili, J. (2013). The role of physical activity in cancer prevention, treatment, recovery, and survivorship. *Oncology, 27,* 580–585. Retrieved from http://www.cancernetwork.com/survivorship/role-physical-activity -cancer-prevention-treatment-recovery-and-survivorship

Ma, H., Xu, X., Clague, J., Lu, Y., Togawa, K., Wang, S.S., … Bernstein, L. (2016). Recreational physical activity and risk of triple negative breast cancer in the California Teachers Study. *Breast Cancer Research, 18,* 62. doi:10.1186/s13058-016 -0723-3

Moore, S.C., Lee, I.-M., Weiderpass, E., Campbell, P.T., Sampson, J.N., Kitahara, C.M., … Patel, A.V. (2016). Association of leisure-time physical activity with risk of 26 types of cancer in 1.44 million adults. *JAMA Internal Medicine, 176,* 816–825. doi:10.1001/jamainternmed.2016.1548

Na, H.-K., & Oliynyk, S. (2011). Effects of physical activity on cancer prevention. *Annals of the New York Academy of Sciences, 1229,* 176–183. doi:10.1111/j.1749 -6632.2011.06105.x

National Cancer Institute. (2017). Physical activity and cancer. Retrieved from https:// www.cancer.gov/about-cancer/causes-prevention/risk/obesity/physical-activity -fact-sheet

National Institutes of Health. (2016). Physical activity and your heart. Retrieved from https://www.nhlbi.nih.gov/book/export/html/4853

Office of Disease Prevention and Health Promotion. (2008). Physical activity guidelines for Americans. Retrieved from https://health.gov/paguidelines /guidelines

Rogers, C.J., Colbert, L.H., Greiner, J.W., Perkins, S.N., & Hursting, S.D. (2008). Physical activity and cancer prevention. *Sports Medicine, 38,* 271–296. doi:10 .2165/00007256-200838040-00002

Schmitz, K.H., Courneya, K.S., Matthews, C., Demark-Wahnefried, W., Galvão, D.A., Pinto, B.M., … Schwartz, A.L. (2010). American College of Sports Medicine round-table on exercise guidelines for cancer survivors. *Medicine and Science in Sports and Exercise, 42,* 1409–1426. doi:10.1249/mss.0b013e3181e0c112

Thomson, C.A., McCullough, M.L., Wertheim, B.C., Chlebowski, R.T., Martinez, M.E., Stefanick, M.L., … Neuhouser, M.L. (2014). Nutrition and physical activity cancer prevention guidelines, cancer risk, and mortality in the women's health initiative. *Cancer Prevention Research, 7,* 42–53. doi:10.1158/1940-6207.capr-13-0258

Walter, R.B., Buckley, S.A., & White, E. (2012). Regular recreational physical activity and risk of hematologic malignancies: Results from the prospective VITamins And lifestyle (VITAL) study. *Annals of Oncology, 24,* 1370–1377. doi:10.1093/annonc /mds631

Winzer, B.M., Whiteman, D.C., Reeves, M.M., & Paratz, J.D. (2011). Physical activity and cancer prevention: A systematic review of clinical trials. *Cancer Causes and Control, 22,* 811–826. doi:10.1007/s10552-011-9761-4

Chapter 5. Food and Nutrition

American Institute for Cancer Research. (n.d.-a). Obesity and cancer risk. Retrieved from   http://www.aicr.org/reduce-your-cancer-risk/weight/reduce_weight_cancer_link.html

American Institute for Cancer Research. (n.d.-b). Recommendations for cancer prevention. Retrieved from http://www.aicr.org/reduce-your-cancer-risk/recommendations-for-cancer-prevention

Byers, T. (2015a, April). *Meta-analysis of over 20 years of research involving over 300,000 people using over-the-counter supplements.* Paper presented at the 2015 American Association for Cancer Research Annual Meeting, Philadelphia, PA.

Byers, T. (2015b, April). *Opening keynote.* Lecture presented at the 2015 American Association for Cancer Research Annual Meeting, Philadelphia, PA.

Centers for Disease Control and Prevention. (2016). National Health Interview Survey. Retrieved from http://www.cdc.gov/nchs/nhis/releases/released201605.htm

Environmental Working Group. (2017). Executive summary: EWG's 2017 Shopper's Guide to Pesticides in Produce™. Retrieved from https://www.ewg.org/foodnews/summary.php

Hardy, T.M., & Tollefsbol, T.O. (2011). Epigenetic diet: Impact on the epigenome and cancer. *Epigenomics, 3,* 503–518. doi:10.2217/epi.11.71

Imayama, I., Ulrich, C.M., Alfano, C.M., Wang, C., Xiao, L., Wener, M.H., ... McTiernan, A. (2012). Effects of a caloric restriction weight loss diet and exercise on inflammatory biomarkers in overweight/obese postmenopausal women: A randomized controlled trial. *Cancer Research, 72,* 2314–2326. doi:10.1158/0008-5472.CAN-11-3092

Jacobs, D.R., Jr., & Steffen, L.M. (2003). Nutrients, foods, and dietary patterns as exposures in research: A framework for food synergy. *American Journal of Clinical Nutrition, 78*(Suppl. 3), 508S–513S.

Katz, R. (2017). *The cancer-fighting kitchen: Nourishing, big-flavor recipes for cancer treatment and recovery.* New York, NY: Ten Speed Press.

Kushi, L.H., Doyle, C., McCullough, M., Rock, C.L., Demark-Wahnefried, W., Bandera, E.V., ... Gansler, T. (2012). American Cancer Society guidelines on nutrition and physical activity for cancer prevention. *CA: A Cancer Journal for Clinicians, 62,* 30–67. doi:10.3322/caac.20140

Lev-Ari, S., Strier, L., Kazanov, D., Madar-Shapiro, L., Dvory-Sobol, H., Pinchuk, I., ... Arber, N. (2005). Celecoxib and curcumin synergistically inhibit the growth of colorectal cancer cells. *Clinical Cancer Research, 11,* 6738–6744. doi:10.1158/1078-0432.CCR-05-017-1

Navarro, V.J., Khan, I., Björnsson, E., Seeff, L.B., Serrano, J., & Hoofnagle, J.H. (2017). Liver injury from herbal and dietary supplements. *Hepatology, 65,* 363–373. doi:10.1002/hep.28813

Nechuta, S.J., Caan, B.J., Chen, W.Y., Lu, W., Chen, Z., Kwan, M.L., ... Shu, X.O. (2012). Soy food intake after diagnosis of breast cancer and survival: An in-depth analysis of combined evidence from cohort studies of US and Chinese women. *American Journal of Clinical Nutrition, 96,* 123–132. doi:10.3945/ajcn.112.035972

Priyadarsini, R.V., & Nagini, S. (2012). Cancer chemoprevention by dietary phytochemicals: Promises and pitfalls. *Current Pharmaceutical Biotechnology, 13,* 125–136.

Samraj, A.N., Pearce, O.M.T., Läubli, H., Crittenden, A.N., Bergfeld, A.K., Banda, K., … Varki, A. (2015). A red meat-derived glycan promotes inflammation and cancer progression. *Proceedings of the National Academy of Sciences of the United States of America, 112,* 542–547. doi:10.1073/pnas.1417508112

Simopoulos, A.P. (2008). The importance of the omega-6/omega-3 fatty acid ratio in cardiovascular disease and other chronic diseases. *Experimental Biology and Medicine, 233,* 674–688. doi:10.3181/0711-MR-311

Sundem, G. (2015, April 20). Dietary supplements shown to increase cancer risk. *Colorado Cancer Blogs.* Retrieved from http://www.coloradocancerblogs.org /dietary-supplements-shown-to-increase-cancer-risk

U.S. Burden of Disease Collaborators. (2013). The state of US health, 1990–2010: Burden of diseases, injuries and risk factors. *JAMA, 310,* 591–608. doi:10.1001 /jama.2013.13805

World Cancer Research Fund & American Institute for Cancer Research. (2007). *Food, nutrition, physical activity, and the prevention of cancer: A global perspective.* Washington, DC: Authors.

Zong, C., Gao, A., Hu, F.B., & Sun, Q. (2016). Whole grain intake and mortality from all causes, cardiovascular disease, and cancer: A meta-analysis of prospective cohort studies. *Circulation, 133,* 2370–2380. doi:10.1161/CIRCULATIONAHA.115.021101

Chapter 6. Alcohol and Tobacco

Allen, N.E., Beral, V., Casabonne, D., Kan, S.W., Reeves, G.K., Brown, A., & Green, J. (2009). Moderate alcohol intake and cancer incidence in women. *Journal of the National Cancer Institute, 101,* 296–305. doi:10.1093/jnci/djn514

American Cancer Society. (2015). Why people start smoking and why it's hard to stop. Retrieved from http://www.cancer.org/cancer/cancercauses/tobaccocancer /why-people-start-using-tobacco

American Heart Association. (2015). Alcohol and heart health. Retrieved from http:// www.heart.org/HEARTORG/Conditions/More/MyHeartandStrokeNews/Alcohol -and-Heart-Disease_UCM_305173_Article.jsp#.V3sK4ZMrKRt

American Liver Foundation. (n.d.). Alcohol related liver disease. Retrieved from http:// www.liverfoundation.org/downloads/alf_download_828.pdf

American Lung Association. (n.d.). COPD. Retrieved from http://www.lung.org/lung -health-and-diseases/lung-disease-lookup/copd

American Lung Association. (2016). What is COPD: Chronic bronchitis and emphysema. Retrieved from http://www.lung.org/lung-health-and-diseases/lung-disease -lookup/copd/learn-about-copd/what-is-copd.html

American Lung Association Research and Program Services, Epidemiology and Statistics Unit. (2011). *Trends in tobacco use.* Retrieved from http://www.lung.org /assets/documents/research/tobacco-trend-report.pdf

Bjartveit, K., & Tverdal, A. (2005). Health consequences of smoking 1–4 cigarettes per day. *Tobacco Control, 14,* 315–320. doi:10.1136/tc.2005.011932

Carrigan, M.A., Uryasev, O., Frye, C.B., Eckman, B.L., Myers, C.R., Hurley, T.D., & Benner, S.A. (2014). Hominids adapted to metabolize ethanol long before human-directed fermentation. *Proceedings of the National Academy of Sciences of the United States of America, 112,* 458–463. doi:10.1073/pnas.1404167111

Dudley, R. (2014). *The drunken monkey: Why we drink and abuse alcohol.* Berkeley, CA: University of California Press.

International Agency for Research on Cancer Working Group on the Evaluation of Carcinogenic Risks to Humans. (2010). *Alcohol consumption and ethyl carbamate.* Retrieved from http://monographs.iarc.fr/ENG/Monographs/vol96/mono96.pdf

National Cancer Institute. (2010). "Light" cigarettes and cancer risk. Retrieved from http://www.cancer.gov/about-cancer/causes-prevention/risk/tobacco/light-cigarettes-fact-sheet

National Cancer Institute. (2013). Alcohol and cancer risk. Retrieved from https://www.cancer.gov/about-cancer/causes-prevention/risk/alcohol/alcohol-fact-sheet

National Cancer Institute. (2014). Harms of cigarette smoking and health benefits of quitting. Retrieved from http://www.cancer.gov/about-cancer/causes-prevention/risk/tobacco/cessation-fact-sheet

National Cancer Institute. (2017). Tobacco. Retrieved from https://www.cancer.gov/about-cancer/causes-prevention/risk/tobacco

National Institute on Alcohol Abuse and Alcoholism. (n.d.-a). Alcohol's effects on the body. Retrieved from https://www.niaaa.nih.gov/alcohol-health/alcohols-effects-body

National Institute on Alcohol Abuse and Alcoholism. (n.d.-b). Drinking levels defined. Retrieved from http://www.niaaa.nih.gov/alcohol-health/overview-alcohol-consumption/moderate-binge-drinking

National Institute on Alcohol Abuse and Alcoholism. (2017). Alcohol facts and statistics. Retrieved from http://pubs.niaaa.nih.gov/publications/AlcoholFacts&Stats/AlcoholFacts&Stats.htm

National Toxicology Program. (2016). *Report on carcinogens* (14th ed.). Retrieved from http://ntp.niehs.nih.gov/go/roc14

Olson, K.N., Smith, S.W., Kloss, J.S., Ho, J.D., & Apple, F.S. (2013). Relationship between blood alcohol concentration and observable symptoms of intoxication in patients presenting to an emergency department. *Alcohol and Alcoholism, 48,* 386–389. doi:10.1093/alcalc/agt042

Parsons, A., Daley, A., Begh, R., & Aveyard, P. (2010). Influence of smoking cessation after diagnosis of early stage lung cancer on prognosis: Systematic review of observational studies with meta-analysis. *BMJ, 340,* b5569. doi:10.1136/bmj.b5569

Qiao, Q., Tervahauta, M., Nissinen, A., & Tuomilehto, J. (2000). Mortality from all causes and from coronary heart disease related to smoking and changes in smoking during a 35-year follow-up of middle-aged Finnish men. *European Heart Journal, 21,* 1621–1626. doi:10.1053/euhj.2000.2151

Randall, V.R. (1999). History of tobacco. Retrieved from http://academic.udayton.edu/health/syllabi/tobacco/history.htm

Taylor, T. (2014, May 29). The drunken monkey: Why we drink and abuse alcohol, by Robert Dudley: Tiffany Taylor on a thought-provoking exploration of alcoholism from an evolutionary perspective [Review]. Retrieved from https://www.timeshighereducation.com/books/the-drunken-monkey-why-we-drink-and-abuse-alcohol-by-robert-dudley/2013542.article

Tolstrup, J.S., Hvidtfeldt, U.A., Flachs, E.M., Spiegelman, D., Heitmann, B.L., Bälter, K., ... Feskanich, D. (2014). Smoking and risk of coronary heart disease in younger, middle-aged, and older adults. *American Journal of Public Health, 104,* 96–102. doi:10.2105/AJPH.2012.301091

U.S. Department of Health and Human Services. (2004). *The health consequences of smoking: A report of the Surgeon General.* Retrieved from https://www.cdc.gov/tobacco/data_statistics/sgr/2004/index.htm

U.S. Department of Health and Human Services. (2014). *The health consequences of smoking—50 years of progress: A report of the Surgeon General.* Retrieved from http://www.surgeongeneral.gov/library/reports/50-years-of-progress/full-report.pdf

Vice. (n.d.). In Dictionary.com. Retrieved from http://www.dictionary.com/browse/vice?s=t

Chapter 7. Viruses and Vaccines

American Cancer Society. (2016). Cancer vaccines. Retrieved from http://www.cancer.org/treatment/treatments-and-side-effects/treatmenttypes/immunotherapy/immunotherapy-cancer-vaccines.html

Cancer.Net Editorial Board. (2016). What are cancer vaccines? Retrieved from http://www.cancer.net/navigating-cancer-care/how-cancer-treated/immunotherapy-and-vaccines/what-are-cancer-vaccines

Centers for Disease Control and Prevention. (2016a). Finding and paying for vaccines. Retrieved from https://www.cdc.gov/vaccines/adults/find-pay-vaccines.html

Centers for Disease Control and Prevention. (2016b). Hepatitis B vaccine: What you need to know. Retrieved from https://www.cdc.gov/vaccines/hcp/vis/vis-statements/hep-b.pdf

Centers for Disease Control and Prevention. (2016c). HPV. Retrieved from http://www.cdc.gov/vaccines/parents/diseases/teen/hpv-indepth-color.pdf

Centers for Disease Control and Prevention. (2017). 2017 recommended immunizations for adults: By age. Retrieved from https://www.cdc.gov/vaccines/schedules/downloads/adult/adult-schedule-easy-read-bw.pdf

Hale, D.F., Vreeland, T.J., & Peoples, G.E. (2016). Arming the immune system through vaccination to prevent cancer recurrence. *American Society of Clinical Oncology Education Book, 35,* e159–e167. Retrieved from http://meetinglibrary.asco.org/collections/edbook/2016%20ASCO%20Educational%20Book

Markowitz, L.E., Dunne, E.F., Saraiya, M., Chesson, H.W., Curtis, C.R., Gee, J., ... Unger, E.R. (2014). Human papillomavirus vaccination: Recommendations of the Advisory Committee on Immunization Practices (ACIP). *MMWR Recommendations and Reports, 63*(RR5), 1–30. Retrieved from http://www.cdc.gov/mmwr/preview/mmwrhtml/rr6305a1.htm

National Institutes of Health. (2017). ClinicalTrials.gov. Retrieved from https://clinicaltrials.gov

National Toxicology Program. (2016). *Report on carcinogens* (14th ed.). Retrieved from http://ntp.niehs.nih.gov/go/roc14

Plummer, M., de Martel, C., Vignat, J., Ferlay, J., Bray, F., & Franceschi, S. (2016). Global burden of cancers attributable to infections in 2012: A synthetic analysis. *Lancet Global Health, 4,* e609–e615. doi:10.1016/S2214-109X(16)30143-7

Viens, L.J., Henley, S.J., Watson, M., Markowitz, L.E., Thomas, C.C., Thompson, T.D., ... Saraiya, M. (2016). Human papillomavirus-associated cancers—United States, 2008–2012. *Morbidity and Mortality Weekly Report, 65,* 661–666. doi:10.15585/mmwr.mm6526a1

World Health Organization. (2016). *Global health sector strategy on viral hepatitis, 2016–2021.* Retrieved from http://www.who.int/hepatitis/strategy2016-2021/ghss-hep/en

World Health Organization. (2017). Hepatitis B. Retrieved from http://www.who.int/mediacentre/factsheets/fs204/en

Chapter 8. Physiologic Stress and Inflammation

American Cancer Society. (2016). Infections that can lead to cancer. Retrieved from https://www.cancer.org/cancer/cancer-causes/infectious-agents/infections-that-can-lead-to-cancer.html

American College of Allergy, Asthma, and Immunology. (2014). Drug allergies. Retrieved from http://acaai.org/allergies/types/drug-allergies

Anderson, R., Tintinger, G.R., & Feldman, C. (2014). Inflammation and cancer: The role of the human neutrophil. *South African Journal of Science, 110*(1/2), 36–41. doi:10.1590/sajs.2014/20130207

Chai, E.Z.P., Siveen, K.S., Shanmugam, M.K., Arfuso, F., & Sethi, G. (2015). Analysis of the intricate relationship between chronic inflammation and cancer. *Biochemical Journal, 468,* 1–15. doi:10.1042/BJ20141337

Elinav, E., Nowarski, R., Thaiss, C.A., Hu, B., Jin, C., & Flavell, R.A. (2013). Inflammation-induced cancer: Crosstalk between tumours, immune cells, and microorganisms. *Nature Reviews Cancer, 13,* 759–771. doi:10.1038/nrc3611

Giugliano, D., Ceriello, A., & Esposito, K. (2006). The effects of diet on inflammation: Emphasis on the metabolic syndrome. *Journal of the American College of Cardiology, 48,* 677–685. doi:10.1016/j.jacc.2006.03.052

Limón-Pacheco, J., & Gonsebatt, M.E. (2009). The role of antioxidants and antioxidant-related enzymes in protective responses to environmentally induced oxidative stress. *Mutation Research/Genetic Toxicology and Environmental Mutagenesis, 674,* 137–147. doi:10.1016/j.mrgentox.2008.09.015

National Cancer Institute. (2014). Antioxidants and cancer prevention. Retrieved from http://www.cancer.gov/about-cancer/causes-prevention/risk/diet/antioxidants-fact-sheet

National Cancer Institute. (2015). Chronic inflammation. Retrieved from http://www.cancer.gov/about-cancer/causes-prevention/risk/chronic-inflammation

National Institutes of Health. (n.d.). *5 things you should know about stress* (NIH Publication No. OM 16-4310). Retrieved from https://www.nimh.nih.gov/health/publications/stress/index.shtml

Porta, C., Larghi, P., Rimoldi, M., Totaro, M.G., Allavena, P., Mantovani, A., & Sica, A. (2009). Cellular and molecular pathways linking inflammation and cancer. *Immunobiology, 214,* 761–777. doi:10.1016/j.imbio.2009.06.014

Reuter, S., Gupta, S.C., Chaturvedi, M.M., & Aggarwal, B.B. (2010). Oxidative stress, inflammation, and cancer: How are they linked? *Free Radical Biology and Medicine, 49,* 1603–1616. doi:10.1016/j.freeradbiomed.2010.09.006

U.S. Environmental Protection Agency. (2017). Our mission and what we do. Retrieved from https://www.epa.gov/aboutepa/our-mission-and-what-we-do

Valente, A.L., Schroeder, B., Shriver, C.D., Henning, J.D., & Ellsworth, R.E. (2015). Chronic inflammation in cancer: The role of human viruses. *Advances in Tumor Virology, 5,* 1–11. doi:10.4137/ATV.S19779

Chapter 9. Radiation Exposure

American Cancer Society. (2015). What are x-rays and gamma rays? Retrieved from https://www.cancer.org/cancer/cancer-causes/radiation-exposure/x-rays-gamma-rays/what-are-xrays-and-gamma-rays.html

American Cancer Society. (2016). Known and probable human carcinogens. Retrieved from https://www.cancer.org/cancer/cancer-causes/general-info/known-and-probable-human-carcinogens.html

American Cancer Society. (2017). What is ultraviolet (UV) radiation? Retrieved from https://www.cancer.org/cancer/skin-cancer/prevention-and-early-detection/what-is-uv-radiation.html

Centers for Disease Control and Prevention. (2016a). Radiation from space (cosmic radiation). Retrieved from http://www.cdc.gov/nceh/radiation/cosmic.html

Centers for Disease Control and Prevention. (2016b). Ultraviolet radiation. Retrieved from https://www.cdc.gov/nceh/radiation/ultraviolet.htm

Daniels, R.D., & Sylvain, D.C. (2012). *Evaluation of exposure to radon progeny during closure of inactive uranium mines—Colorado* (NIOSH HETA No. 2011-0090-3161). Retrieved from https://www.cdc.gov/niosh/hhe/reports/pdfs/2011-0090-3161.pdf

Folley, J.H., Borges, W., & Yamawaki, T. (1952). Incidence of leukemia in survivors of the atom bomb in Hiroshima and Nagasaki, Japan. *American Journal of Medicine, 13,* 311–321.

Gale, R.P., & Hoffman, F.O. (2013). Communicating cancer risk from radiation exposures: Nuclear accidents, total body radiation and diagnostic procedures. *Bone Marrow Transplantation, 48,* 2–3. doi:10.1038/bmt.2012.90

Gilbert, E.S. (2009). Ionizing radiation and cancer risks: What have we learned from epidemiology? *International Journal of Radiation Biology, 85,* 467–482. doi:10.1080/09553000902883836

Krewski, D., Lubin, J.H., Zielinski, J.M., Alavanja, M., Catalan, V.S., Field, R.W., ... Wilcox, H.B. (2005). Residential radon and risk of lung cancer: A combined analysis of 7 North American case-control studies. *Epidemiology, 16,* 137–145.

National Cancer Institute. (2017). Sunlight. Retrieved from http://www.cancer.gov/about-cancer/causes-prevention/risk/sunlight

National Institute of Occupational Safety and Health. (2016). Sun exposure. Retrieved from http://www.cdc.gov/niosh/topics/sunexposure/default.html

Preston, D.L., Ron, E., Tokuoka, S., Funamoto, S., Nishi, N., Soda, M., ... Kodama, K. (2007). Solid cancer incidence in atomic bomb survivors: 1958–98. *Radiation Research, 168,* 1–64. doi:10.1667/RR0763.1

Tinney, V. (2014). Children's health and the environment. *The Pennsylvania Nurse, 69*(1), 4–12.

U.S. Environmental Protection Agency. (2016). *A citizen's guide to radon: The guide to protecting yourself and your family from radon.* Retrieved from https://www.epa.gov/sites/production/files/2016-12/documents/2016_a_citizens_guide_to_radon.pdf

U.S. Environmental Protection Agency. (2017a). Health risk of radon. Retrieved from https://www.epa.gov/radon/health-risk-radon

U.S. Environmental Protection Agency. (2017b). Radiation basics. Retrieved from https://www.epa.gov/radiation/radiation-basics

U.S. Food and Drug Administration. (2017). What are the radiation risks from CT? Retrieved from http://www.fda.gov/Radiation-EmittingProducts/RadiationEmittingProductsandProcedures/MedicalImaging/MedicalX-Rays/ucm115329.htm

U.S. Nuclear Regulatory Commission. (2014). Minimize your exposure. Retrieved from http://www.nrc.gov/about-nrc/radiation/protects-you/protection-principles.html

World Health Organization. (n.d.). What is ionizing radiation? Retrieved from http://www.who.int/ionizing_radiation/about/what_is_ir/en

Chapter 10. Genetics

Jacobs, C., Webb, P., & Robinson, L. (2014). *Genetics for health professionals in cancer care: From principles to practice.* Oxford, England: Oxford University Press.

Lister Hill National Center for Biomedical Communications. (2017). *Help me understand genetics.* Retrieved from https://ghr.nlm.nih.gov/primer

Matloff, E.T. (2013). *Cancer principles and practice of oncology: Handbook of clinical cancer genetics.* Philadelphia, PA: Lippincott Williams & Wilkins.

MedlinePlus. (2017). Genetic counseling. Retrieved from https://medlineplus.gov/geneticcounseling.html

National Genetics and Genomics Education Centre. (n.d.). Telling stories: Understanding real life genetics. Retrieved from http://www.tellingstories.nhs.uk

National Human Genome Research Institute. (2015). Genetic Information Nondiscrimination Act of 2008. Retrieved from https://www.genome.gov/10002328

National Society of Genetic Counselors. (n.d.). Genetic counselors. Retrieved from http://aboutgeneticcounselors.com

Schneider, K.A. (2012). *Counseling about cancer: Strategies for genetic counseling* (3rd ed.). Hoboken, NJ: Wiley-Blackwell.

Chapter 11. Cancer and the Environment

Agency for Toxic Substances and Disease Registry. (2016). Asbestos toxicity: What respiratory conditions are associated with asbestos? Retrieved from http://www.atsdr.cdc.gov/csem/csem.asp?csem=29&po=11

Alexander, D.D., Weed, D.L., Mink, P.J., & Mitchell, M.E. (2012). A weight-of-evidence review of colorectal cancer in pesticide applicators: The agricultural health study and other epidemiologic studies. *International Archives of Occupational and Environmental Health, 85,* 715–745. doi:10.1007/s00420-011-0723-7

American Cancer Society. (2014). Antiperspirants and breast cancer risk. Retrieved from https://www.cancer.org/cancer/cancer-causes/antiperspirants-and-breast-cancer-risk.html

American Cancer Society. (2015a). Asbestos and cancer risk. Retrieved from https://www.cancer.org/cancer/cancer-causes/asbestos.html

American Cancer Society. (2015b). Radon and cancer. Retrieved from https://www.cancer.org/cancer/cancer-causes/radiation-exposure/radon.html

American Cancer Society. (2016). Benzene and cancer risk. Retrieved from https://www.cancer.org/cancer/cancer-causes/benzene.html?sitearea=PED

American Cancer Society. (2017). Talcum powder and cancer. Retrieved from https://www.cancer.org/cancer/cancer-causes/talcum-powder-and-cancer.html

American Federation of Teachers. (2010). Hazard circle chart. Retrieved from https://www.osha.gov/dte/grant_materials/fy10/sh-20839-10.html

Anjum, B., Singh, R.B., Verma, N., Singh, R., Mahdi, A.A., Singh, R.K., ... Wilson, D.W. (2012). Associations of circadian disruption of sleep and nutritional factors with risk of cancer. *Open Nutraceuticals Journal, 5,* 124–135. doi:10.2174/1876396001205010124

Anna, D.H. (Ed.). (2011). *Occupational environment: Its evaluation, control and management* (3rd ed., Vol. 1). Falls Church, VA: American Industrial Hygiene Association.

Aronson, K.J., Grundy, A., Korsiak, J., & Spinelli, J.J. (2015). Causes of breast cancer: Could work at night really be a cause? *Breast Cancer Management, 4,* 125–127. doi:10.2217/bmt.15.4

Asbestos.com. (2016). Asbestos, 9/11 and the World Trade Center. Retrieved from https://www.asbestos.com/world-trade-center

Boffetta, P. (2006). Human cancer from environmental pollutants: The epidemiological evidence. *Mutation Research/Genetic Toxicology and Environmental Mutagenesis, 608,* 157–162. doi:10.1016/j.mrgentox.2006.02.015

Boice, J.D., Jr., Blettner, M., & Auvinen, A. (2000). Epidemiologic studies of pilots and aircrew. *Health Physics, 79,* 576–584.

Breastcancer.org. (n.d.-a). Exposure to chemicals in cosmetics. Retrieved from http://www.breastcancer.org/risk/factors/cosmetics

Breastcancer.org. (n.d.-b). Exposure to chemicals in water. Retrieved from http://www.breastcancer.org/risk/factors/water_chem

Budnik, L.T., Kloth, S., Velasco-Garrido, M., & Baur, X. (2012). Prostate cancer and toxicity from critical use exemptions of methyl bromide: Environmental protection helps protect against human health risks. *Environmental Health, 11,* 5. doi:10.1186/1476-069x-11-5

Daniels, R.D., Bertke, S., Dahm, M.M., Yiin, J.H., Kubale, T.L., Hales, T.R., … Pinkerton, L.E. (2015). Exposure-response relationships for select cancer and non-cancer health outcomes in a cohort of US firefighters from San Francisco, Chicago and Philadelphia (1950–2009). *Occupational and Environmental Medicine, 72,* 699–706. doi:10.1136/oemed-2014-102671

Davis, S.R., Tao, X., Bernacki, E.J., Alfriend, A.S., & Delowery, M.E. (2013). Evaluation of a bladder cancer cluster in a population of criminal investigators with the Bureau of Alcohol, Tobacco, Firearms and Explosives—Part 2: The association of cancer risk and fire scene investigation. *Journal of Environmental and Public Health, 2013,* 986023. doi:10.1155/2013/986023

Division of Cancer Epidemiology and Genetics, National Cancer Institute. (n.d.). Drinking water contaminants. Retrieved from http://dceg.cancer.gov/research/what-we-study/environment/drinking-water-contaminants

Doheny, K. (2008). Drugs in our drinking water? Retrieved from http://www.webmd.com/a-to-z-guides/features/drugs-in-our-drinking-water#1

Dranitsaris, G., Johnston, M., Poirier, S., Schueller, T., Milliken, D., Green, E., & Zanke, B. (2005). Are health care providers who work with cancer drugs at an increased risk for toxic events? A systematic review and meta-analysis of the literature. *Journal of Oncology Pharmacy Practice, 11,* 69–78.

Fritschi, L., Glass, D.C., Heyworth, J.S., Aronson, K., Girschik, J., Boyle, T., … Erren, T.C. (2011). Hypotheses for mechanisms linking shiftwork and cancer. *Medical Hypotheses, 77,* 430–436. doi:10.1016/j.mehy.2011.06.002

Griffiths, R.F., & Powell, D.M. (2012). The occupational health and safety of flight attendants. *Aviation, Space, and Environmental Medicine, 83,* 514–521.

Gwini, S., MacFarlane, E., Del Monaco, A., McLean, D., Pisaniello, D., Benke, G.P., & Sim, M.R. (2012). Cancer incidence, mortality, and blood lead levels among workers exposed to inorganic lead. *Annals of Epidemiology, 22,* 270–276. doi:10.1016/j.annepidem.2012.01.003

Hamra, G.B., Laden, F., Cohen, A.J., Raaschou-Nielsen, O., Brauer, M., & Loomis, D. (2015). Lung cancer and exposure to nitrogen dioxide and traffic: A systematic review and meta-analysis. *Environmental Health Perspectives, 123,* 1107–1112. doi:10.1289/ehp.1408882

Ide, C.W. (2014). Cancer incidence and mortality in serving whole-time Scottish fire-fighters 1984–2005. *Occupational Medicine, 64,* 421–427. doi:10.1093/occmed/kqu080

International Agency for Research on Cancer. (2012). Soot, as found in occupational exposure of chimney sweeps. In *IARC Monographs on the Evaluation of Carcinogenic Risks to Humans: Vol. 100F. Chemical agents and related occupations* (pp. 209–214). Retrieved from http://monographs.iarc.fr/ENG/Monographs/vol100F/mono100F-21.pdf

Iwatsubo, Y., Bénézet, L., Boutou-Kempf, O., Févotte, J., Garras, L., Goldberg, M., ... Imbernon, E. (2014). An extensive epidemiological investigation of a kidney cancer cluster in a chemical plant: What have we learned? *Occupational and Environmental Medicine, 7,* 4–11. doi:10.1136/oemed-2013-101477

Jemal, A., Center, M.M., DeSantis, C., & Ward, E.M. (2010). Global patterns of cancer incidence and mortality rates and trends. *Cancer Epidemiology, Biomarkers and Prevention, 19,* 1893–1907. doi:10.1158/1055-9965.epi-10-0437

Kennedy, A.L. (2017). The effects of soil pollutants on humans. Retrieved from http://www.livestrong.com/article/176005-the-effects-of-soil-pollution-on-humans

Langhoff, M.D., Kragh-Thomsen, M.B., Stanislaus, S., & Weinreich, U.M. (2014). Almost half of women with malignant mesothelioma were exposed to asbestos at home through their husbands or sons. *Danish Medical Journal, 61,* A4902.

Levy, M., & Leclerc, B.-S. (2012). Fluoride in drinking water and osteosarcoma incidence rates in the continental United States among children and adolescents. *Cancer Epidemiology, 36,* e83–e88. doi:10.1016/j.canep.2011.11.008

Lewis-Mikhael, A.-M., Bueno-Cavanillas, A., Ofir Guiron, T., Olmedo-Requena, R., Delgado-Rodríguez, M., & Jiménez-Moléon, J.J. (2016). Occupational exposure to pesticides and prostate cancer: A systematic review and meta-analysis. *Occupational and Environmental Medicine, 73,* 134–144. doi:10.1136/oemed-2014-102692

Lewis-Mikhael, A.-M., Olmedo-Requena, R., Martínez-Ruiz, V., Bueno-Cavanillas, A., & Jiménez-Moléon, J.J. (2015). Organochlorine pesticides and prostate cancer, is there an association? A meta-analysis of epidemiological evidence. *Cancer Causes and Control, 26,* 1375–1392. doi:10.1007/s10552-015-0643-z

Lie, J.-A.S., Andersen, A., & Kjaerheim, K. (2007). Cancer risk among 43000 Norwegian nurses. *Scandinavian Journal of Work, Environment and Health, 33,* 66–73.

Lundström, N.-G., Englyst, V., Gerhardsson, L., Jin, T., & Nordberg, G. (2006). Lung cancer development in primary smelter workers: A nested case-referent study. *Journal of Occupational and Environmental Medicine, 48,* 376–380. doi:10.1097/01.jom.0000201556.95982.95

Manuwald, U., Velasco Garrido, M., Berger, J., Manz, A., & Baur, X. (2012). Mortality study of chemical workers exposed to dioxins: Follow-up 23 years after chemical plant closure. *Occupational and Environmental Medicine, 69,* 636–642. doi:10.1136/oemed-2012-100682

Mercola, J. (2008). How safe are green cleaning products? Retrieved from http://articles.mercola.com/sites/articles/archive/2008/05/24/how-safe-are-green-cleaning-products.aspx

Mesothelioma Center. (n.d.). Mesothelioma symptoms. Retrieved from http://www.mesotheliomacenter.org/about/mesothelioma-symptoms.php

National Cancer Institute. (2013). Alcohol and cancer risk. Retrieved from https://www.cancer.gov/about-cancer/causes-prevention/risk/alcohol/alcohol-fact-sheet

National Cancer Institute. (2015). Environmental carcinogens and cancer risk. Retrieved from https://www.cancer.gov/about-cancer/causes-prevention/risk /substances/carcinogens

National Cancer Institute. (2016a). Hair dyes and cancer risk. Retrieved from https://www.cancer.gov/about-cancer/causes-prevention/risk/myths/hair -dyes-fact-sheet

National Cancer Institute. (2016b). Interactive maps. State cancer profiles. Retrieved from https://statecancerprofiles.cancer.gov/map/map.noimage.php

National Cancer Institute. (2017). Asbestos exposure and cancer risk. Retrieved from http://www.cancer.gov/about-cancer/causes-prevention/risk/substances/asbestos /asbestos-fact-sheet

National Institute of Environmental Health Sciences. (2003). Cancer and the environment: What you need to know, what you can do (NIH Publication No. 03-2039). Retrieved from https://www.niehs.nih.gov/health/materials/cancer_and_the _environment_508.pdf

National Toxicology Program. (2016). Report on carcinogens (14th ed.). Retrieved from http://ntp.niehs.nih.gov/go/roc14

Oberoi, S., Barchowsky, A., & Wu, F. (2014). The global burden of disease for skin, lung, and bladder cancer caused by arsenic in food. Cancer Epidemiology, Biomarkers and Prevention, 23, 1187–1194. doi:10.1158/1055-9965.epi-13-1317

Olsson, A.C., Xu, Y., Schüz, J., Vlaanderen, J., Kromhout, H., Vermeulen, R., ... Straif, K. (2013). Lung cancer risk among hairdressers: A pooled analysis of case-control studies conducted between 1985 and 2010. American Journal of Epidemiology, 178, 1355–1365. doi:10.1093/aje/kwt119

Quach, T., Doan-Billing, P.A., Layefsky, M., Nelson, D., Nguyen, K.D., Okahara, L., ... Reynolds, P. (2010). Cancer incidence in female cosmetologists and manicurists in California, 1988–2005. American Journal of Epidemiology, 172, 691–699. doi:10.1093/aje/kwq190

Ragin, C., Davis-Reyes, B., Tadesse, H., Daniels, D., Bunker, C.H., Jackson, M., ... Taioli, E. (2013). Farming, reported pesticide use, and prostate cancer. American Journal of Men's Health, 7, 102–109. doi:10.1177/1557988312458792

Reuben, S.H. (2010). Reducing environmental cancer risk: What we can do now. Retrieved from http://deainfo.nci.nih.gov/advisory/pcp/annualReports/pcp08-09rpt /PCP_Report_08-09_508.pdf

Reynolds, P., Cone, J., Layefsky, M., Goldberg, D.E., & Hurley, S. (2002). Cancer incidence in California flight attendants (United States). Cancer Causes and Control, 13, 317–324.

Robinson, C.F., Sullivan, P.A., Li, J., & Walker, J.T. (2011). Occupational lung cancer in US women, 1984–1998. American Journal of Industrial Medicine, 54, 102–117. doi:10.1002/ajim.20905

Schinasi, L.H., De Roos, A.J., Ray, R.M., Edlefsen, K.L., Parks, C.G., Howard, B.V., ... LaCroix, A.Z. (2015). Insecticide exposure and farm history in relation to risk of lymphomas and leukemias in the Women's Health Initiative observational study cohort. Annals of Epidemiology, 25, 803–810. doi:10.1016/j.annepidem.2015.08 .002

Schinasi, L.H., & Leon, M.E. (2014). Non-Hodgkin lymphoma and occupational exposure to agricultural pesticide chemical groups and active ingredients: A systematic review and meta-analysis [Supplemental material]. International Journal of Environmental Research and Public Health, 11, 4449–4527. doi:10.3390/ijerph110404449

Schottenfeld, D., Beebe-Dimmer, J.L., Buffler, P.A., & Omenn, G.S. (2013). Current perspective on the global and United States cancer burden attributable to lifestyle and environmental risk factors. *Annual Review of Public Health, 34,* 97–117. doi:10.1146/annurev-publhealth-031912-114350

Shay, J.W., Cucinotta, F.A., Sulzman, F.M., Coleman, C.N., & Minna, J.D. (2011). From mice and men to earth and space: Joint NASA-NCI workshop on lung cancer risk resulting from space and terrestrial radiation. *Cancer Research, 71,* 6926–6929. doi:10.1158/0008-5472.can-11-2546

Siegel, R.L., Miller, K.D., & Jemal, A. (2015). Cancer statistics, 2015. *CA: A Cancer Journal for Clinicians, 65,* 5–29. doi:10.3322/caac.21254

Simon, S. (2013). World Health Organization: Outdoor air pollution causes cancer. Retrieved from https://www.cancer.org/latest-news/world-health-organization -outdoor-air-pollution-causes-cancer.html

Stevens, R.G., Hansen, J., Costa, G., Haus, E., Kauppinen, T., Aronson, K.J., ... Straif, K. (2011). Considerations of circadian impact for defining 'shift work' in cancer studies: IARC Working Group report. *Occupational and Environmental Medicine, 68,* 154–162. doi:10.1136/oem.2009.053512

Straif, K., Baan, R., Grosse, Y., Secretan, B., El Ghissassi, F., Bouvard, V., ... Cogliano, V. (2007). Carcinogenicity of shift-work, painting, and fire-fighting. *Lancet Oncology, 8,* 1065–1066. doi:10.1016/S1470-2045(07)70373-X

Sugiura, S., Yagyu, K., Obata, Y., Lin, Y., Tamakoshi, A., Ito, H., ... Kikuchi, S. (2009). Cancer deaths in a cohort of Japanese barbers in Aichi Prefecture. *Asian Pacific Journal of Cancer Prevention, 10,* 307–310.

Torre, L.A., Siegel, R.L., Ward, E.M., & Jemal, A. (2016). Global cancer incidence and mortality rates and trends—An update. *Cancer Epidemiology, Biomarkers and Prevention, 25,* 16–27. doi:10.1158/1055-9965.epi-15-0578

Torres-Durán, M., Ruano-Ravina, A., Parente-Lamelas, I., Leiro-Fernández, V., Abal-Arca, J., Montero-Martínez, C., ... Barros-Dios, J.M. (2015). Residential radon and lung cancer characteristics in never smokers. *International Journal of Radiation Biology, 91,* 605–610. doi:10.3109/09553002.2015.1047985

Tsai, R.J., Luckhaupt, S.E., Schumacher, P., Cress, R.D., Deapen, D.M., & Calvert, G.M. (2015). Risk of cancer among firefighters in California, 1988–2007. *American Journal of Industrial Medicine, 58,* 715–729. doi:10.1002/ajim.22466

U.S. Department of Health and Human Services. (2006). *The health consequences of involuntary exposure to tobacco smoke: A report of the Surgeon General.* Retrieved from http://www.surgeongeneral.gov/library/reports/secondhandsmoke /fullreport.pdf

U.S. Environmental Protection Agency. (2016a). About private water wells. Retrieved from https://www.epa.gov/privatewells/about-private-water-wells

U.S. Environmental Protection Agency. (2016b). *A citizen's guide to radon: The guide to protecting yourself and your family from radon.* Retrieved from https://www.epa .gov/sites/production/files/2016-12/documents/2016_a_citizens_guide_to_radon .pdf

U.S. Environmental Protection Agency. (2017a). Granite countertops and radiation. Retrieved from https://www.epa.gov/radiation/granite-countertops-and-radiation

U.S. Environmental Protection Agency. (2017b). Protect your family. Retrieved from https://www.epa.gov/asbestos/protect-your-family

U.S. Environmental Protection Agency. (2017c). Superfund cleanup process. Retrieved from https://www.epa.gov/superfund/superfund-cleanup-process

Vlaanderen, J., Straif, K., Martinsen, J.I., Kauppinen, T., Pukkla, E., Sparén, P., ... Kjaerheim, K. (2013). Cholangiocarcinoma among workers in the printing industry: Using the Nordic Occupational Cancer database to elucidate a cluster report from Japan. *Occupational and Environmental Medicine, 70*(Suppl. 1), A95.

White, A.J., Teitelbaum, S.L., Stellman, S.D., Beyea, J., Steck, S.E., Mordukhovich, I., ... Gammon, M.D. (2014). Indoor air pollution exposure from use of indoor stoves and fireplaces in association with breast cancer: A case-control study. *Environmental Health, 13,* 108. doi:10.1186/1476-069X-13-108

World Health Organization. (n.d.-a). Ambient air pollution. Retrieved from http://www.who.int/gho/phe/outdoor_air_pollution/en

World Health Organization. (n.d.-b). Fact sheets: Environmental health. Retrieved from http://www.who.int/topics/environmental_health/factsheets/en

World Health Organization. (n.d.-c). Skin cancers. Retrieved from http://www.who.int/uv/faq/skincancer/en/index1.html

World Health Organization. (2011). *An overview of the evidence of the environmental and occupational determinants of cancer.* Presented at WHO First International Conference on Environmental and Occupational Determinants of Cancer: Interventions for Primary Prevention, Asturias, Spain. Retrieved from http://www.who.int/phe/news/events/international_conference/Background_science.pdf

World Health Organization. (2016). Air pollution levels rising in many of the world's poorest cities. Retrieved from http://www.who.int/mediacentre/news/releases/2016/air-pollution-rising/en

Zota, A.R., Aschengrau, A., Rudel, R.A., & Brody, J.G. (2010). Self-reported chemicals exposure, beliefs about disease causation, and risk of breast cancer in the Cape Cod Breast Cancer and Environment Study: A case-control study. *Environmental Health, 9,* 40. doi:10.1186/1476-069X-9-40